Marine Therapy: Health Benefits of Seawater Minerals

All about the natural healing properties of the ocean.

Jose A. Soto, M.D.

AuthorHouse™
1663 Liberty Drive, Suite 200
Bloomington, IN 47403
www.authorhouse.com
Phone: 1-800-839-8640

First published by AuthorHouse12/10/2008

ISBN: 978-1-4389-1974-4 (sc)

Library of Congress Control Number: 2008910495

Printed in the United States of America
Bloomington, Indiana

This book is printed on acid-free paper.

authorHOUSE®

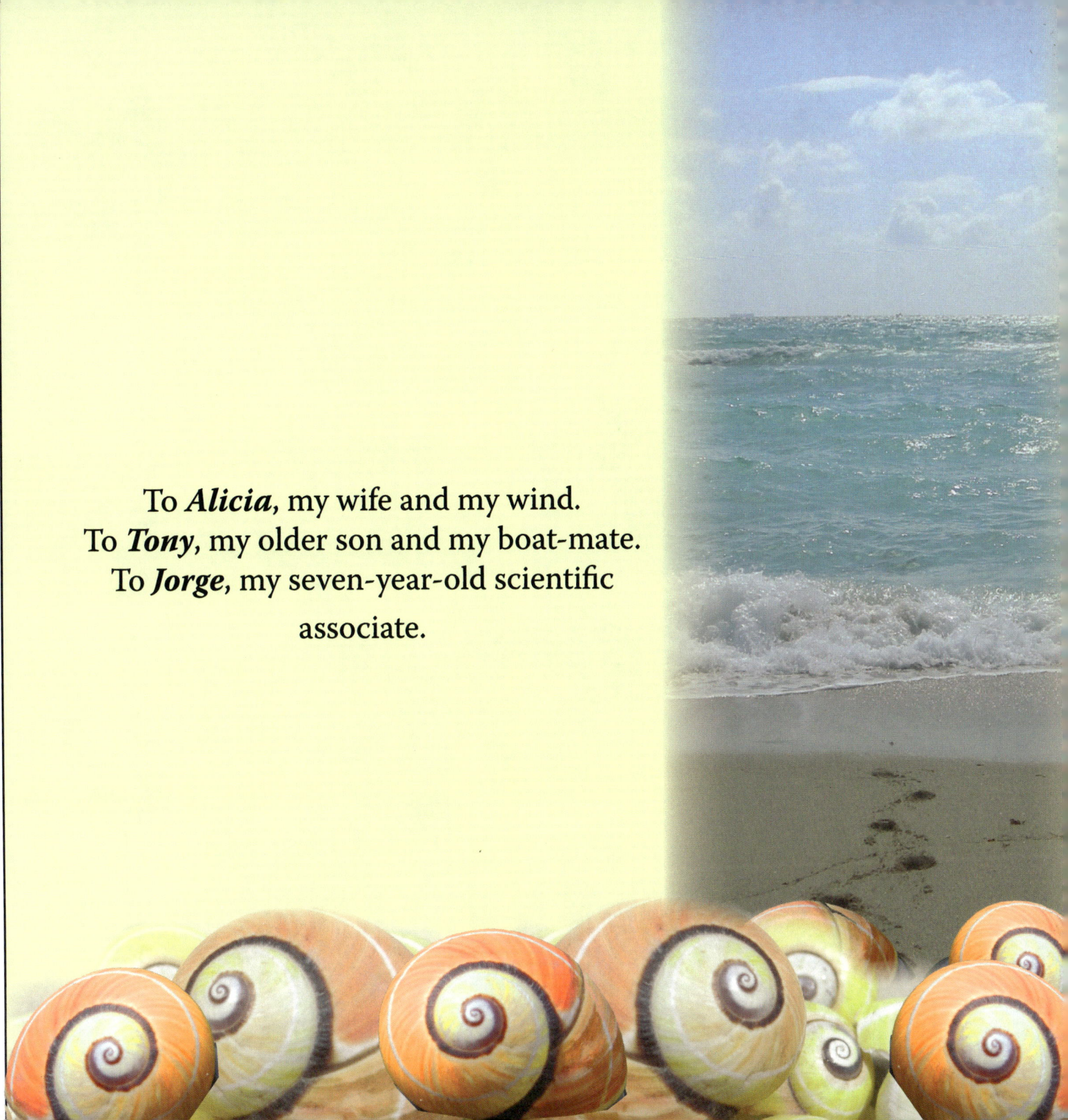

To ***Alicia***, my wife and my wind.
To ***Tony***, my older son and my boat-mate.
To ***Jorge***, my seven-year-old scientific
associate.

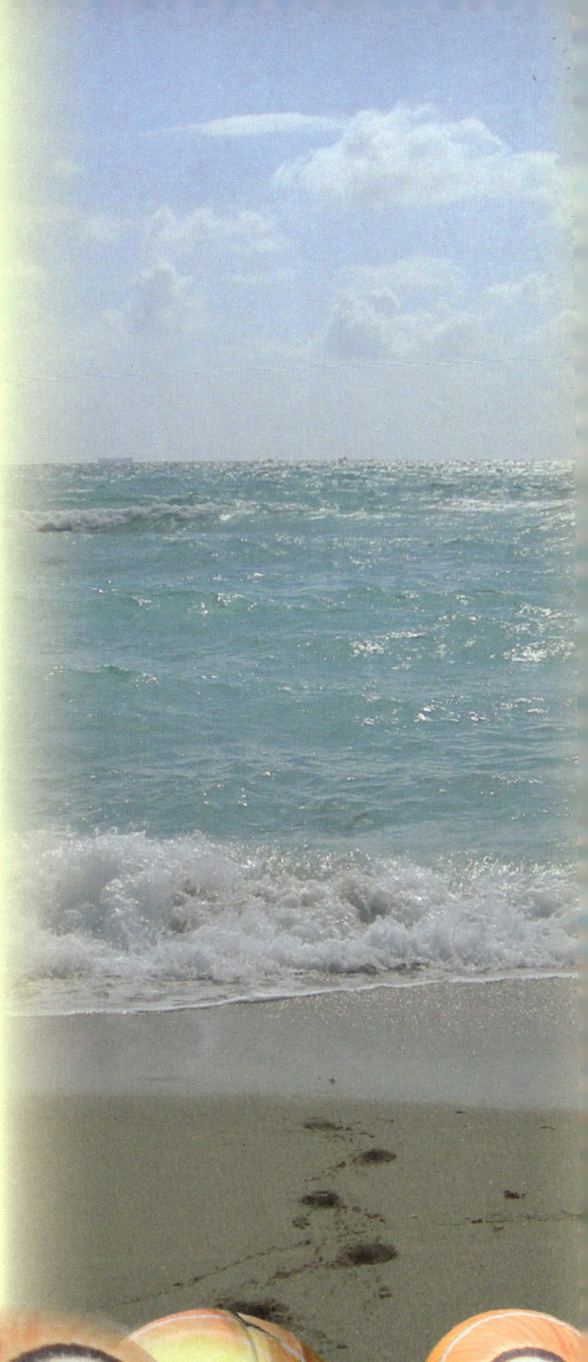

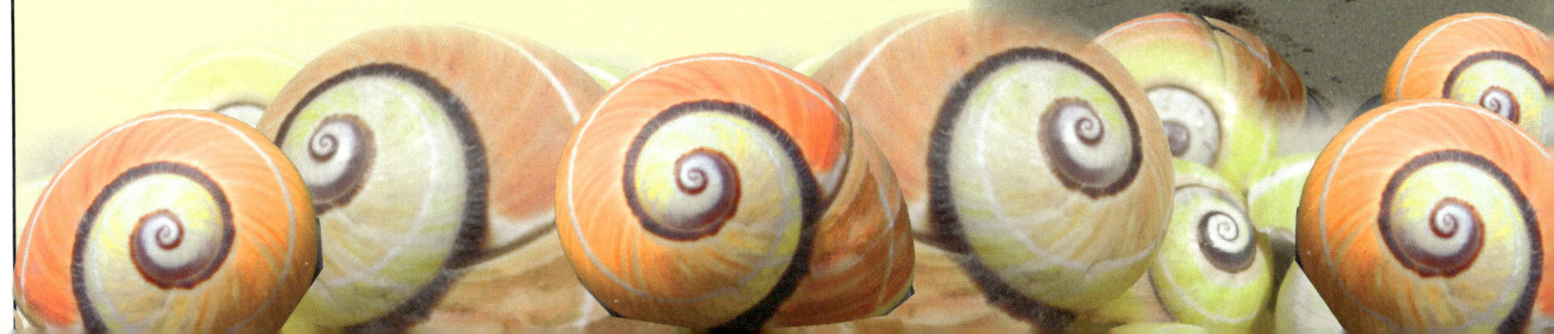

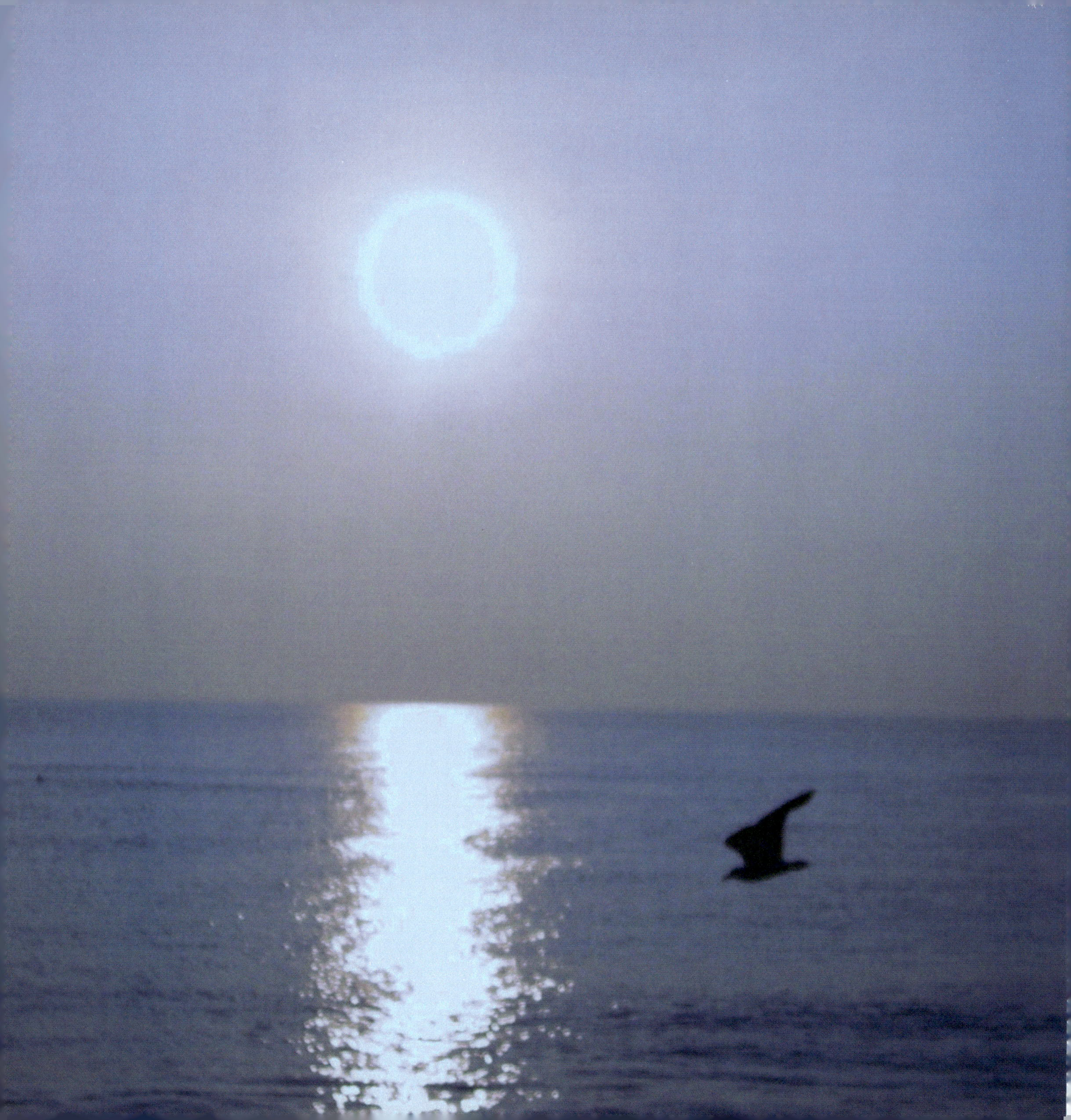

About the Author

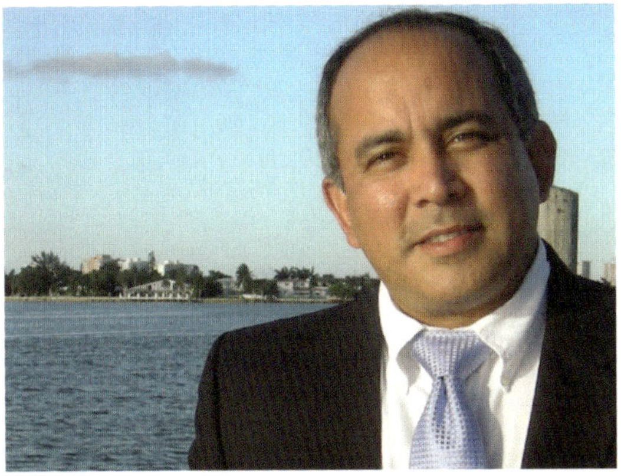

Dr. Jose Antonio Soto, M.D. was born in 1963 near the shores of the Caribbean Sea. He obtained his medical degree in Havana, Cuba, in 1987. The same year he practiced medicine in rural Ethiopia, as part of the world humanitarian help efforts. Dr. Soto emigrated to the United States of America in 1992, and later trained in family medicine at the University of Miami/Jackson Memorial Hospital. He has coursed studies in Harvard and has published more than thirty articles covering diverse scientific aspects and health education topics in Cuba, Mexico, the United States, and Germany. He was granted a patent in 2006 by the United States Patent and Trademark Office in relation to his discovery of the uses of purified ocean water for the treatment of respiratory diseases. He is a member of the American Medical Association and the Society of Cosmetic Chemists. His medical private practice is located in Miami, near Sunny Isles Beach, Florida. He is affiliated with community hospitals in the Miami area. Dr. Soto is a Reuter's insight consultant for medical affairs. His discovery of using seawater for cosmetic and therapeutic purposes has been documented and published in the *International Journal of Applied Sciences,* in Europe, and on the local Fox Network affiliated Channel 7 WSVN, in Miami. He is married and has two children. His main hobby is boating.

Dr. Soto can be contacted at (305) 940-5007 or by e-mail at theoceancure@usa.com His website is www.sea-maronline.com

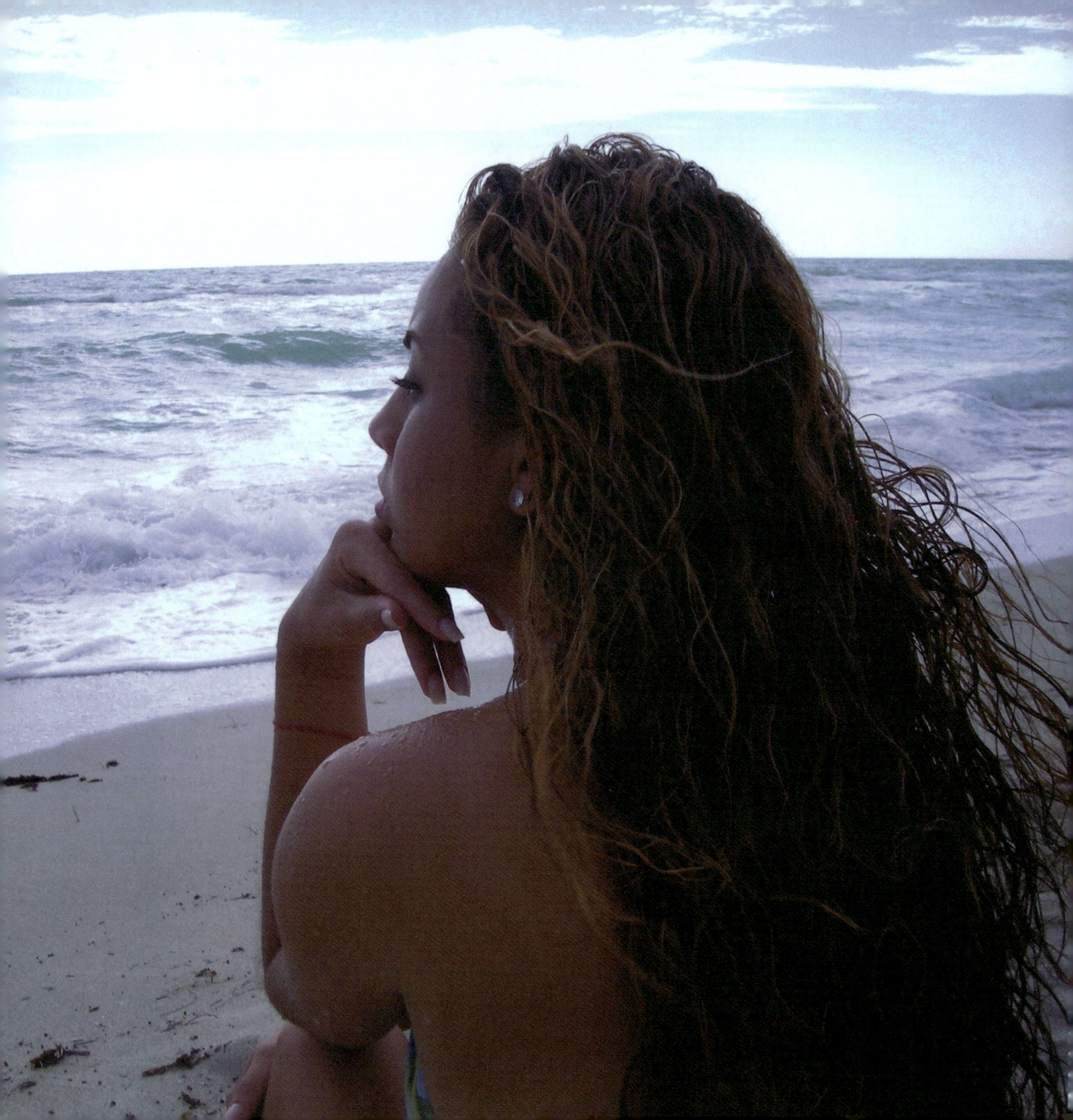

Table of Contents

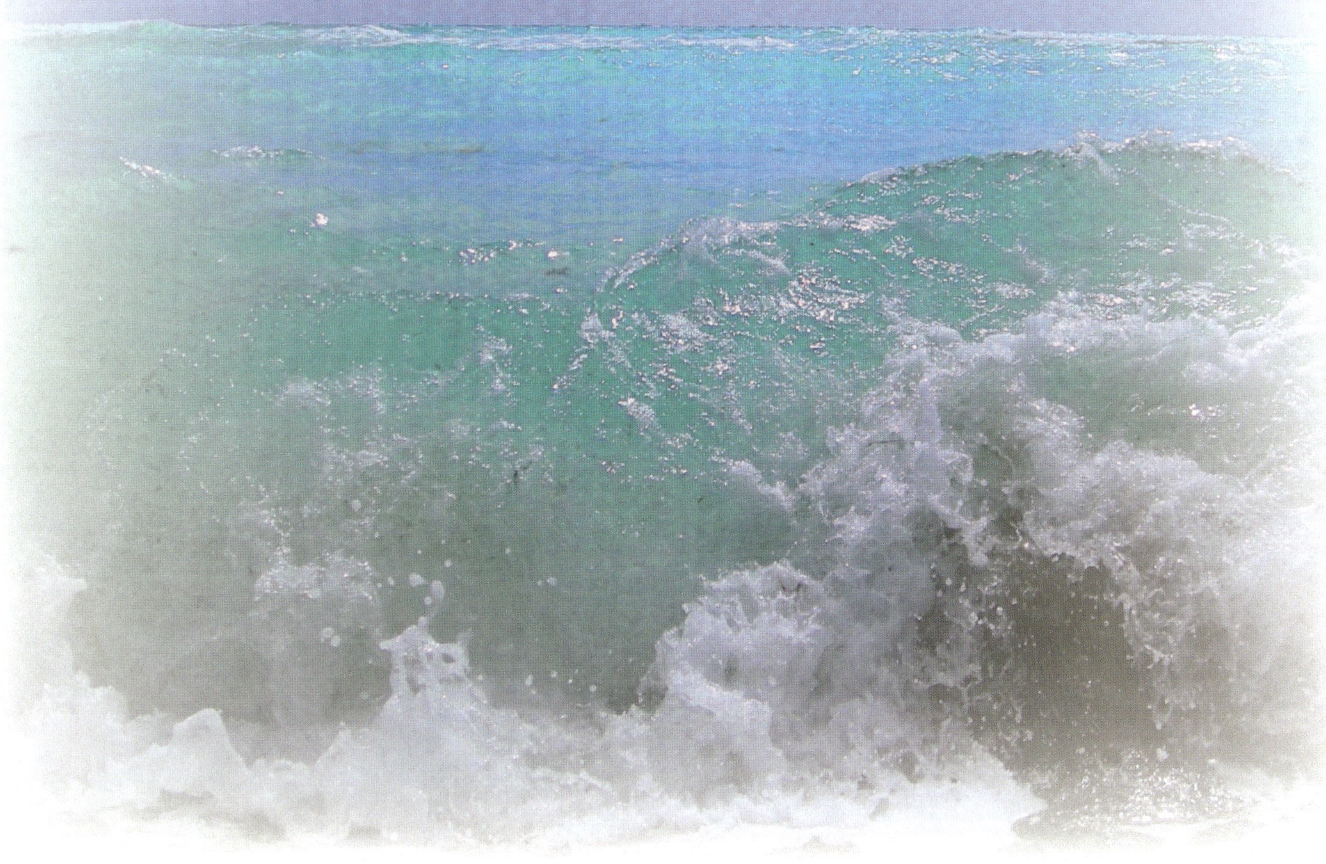

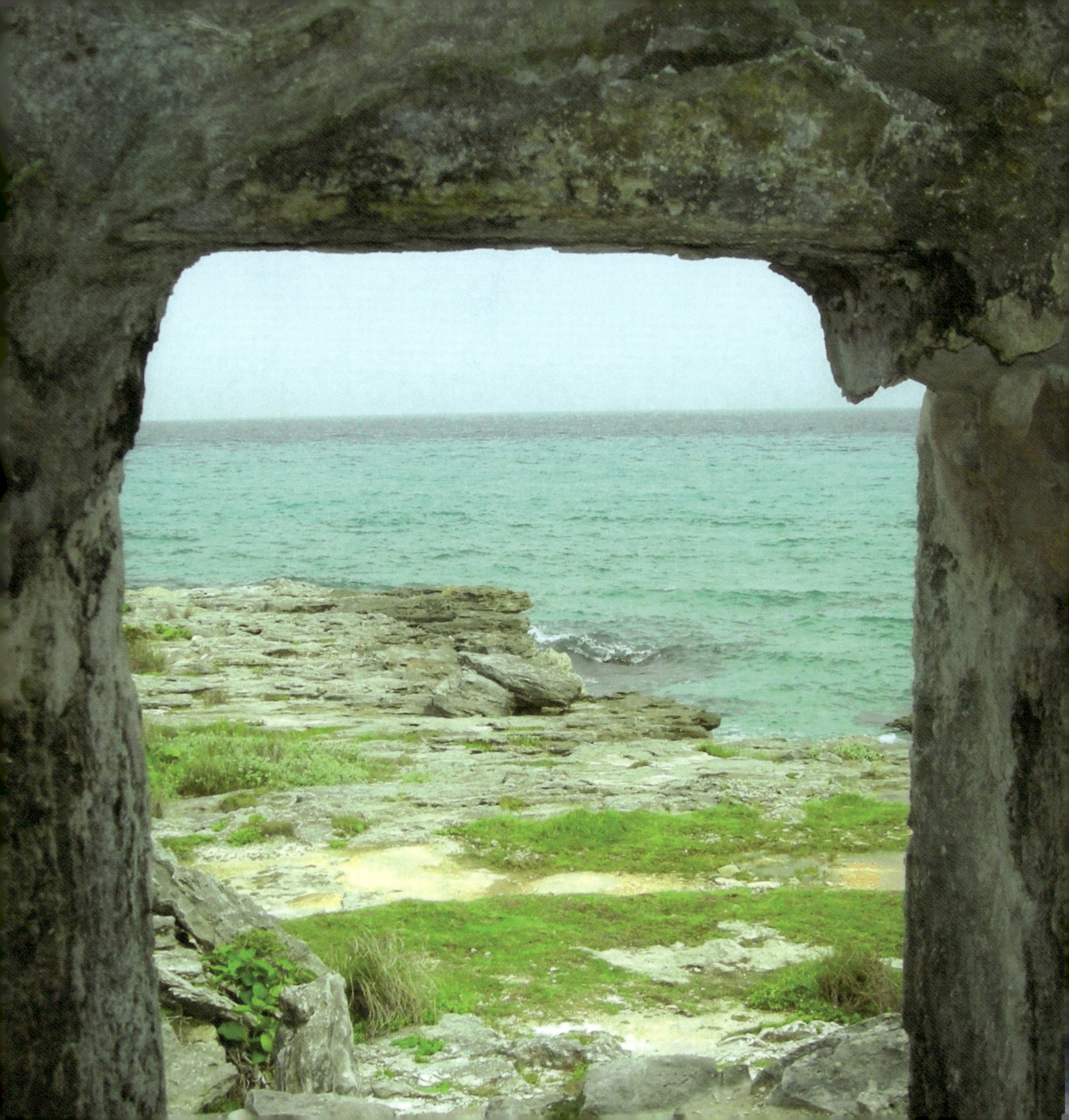

Introduction: Credo and Short Story

My passion for the ocean has its origins from my childhood, on an island that was home to "The Old Man and the Sea." I wouldn't have a perfect vacation unless I was splashing in water by the coast, with my friends, under the vigilant eye of my grandpa. The whole trip to the beach was a fascinating adventure itself—the marine creatures found by the shores, the shells, the algae, and the unforgivable sand in the toes. A burning Caribbean sun was always there, long before global warming, but also there was always plenty of ocean water to play in and refresh our younger bodies.

Beyond the water was the rest of a planet that someone wisely suggested should be called "Planet Ocean" or "Planet Sea." Seventy percent of the earth's surface is covered by an immense sea that was the matrix of all living forms known today. The ocean contains all the natural elements described in the periodic table. Most of the ocean floors are unexplored, and millions of living forms remain unclassified. The ocean is the main source of the oxygen we breathe. The living plankton provides about 80 percent of the oxygen in the atmosphere. The sea was beautiful and powerful, yet deceptive if used to quench a beach boy's thirst. The ocean was always a mystery. The more you read about the ocean, the more you learn, and the more questions arise. New findings bring new hopes.

I decided to pursue this passion years after I graduated from medical school. Everything significantly important in terms of diplomas or licenses was achieved by then. I finished my years of social services in Ethiopia and Cuba. Then I completed my training in family medicine at the University of Miami, Jackson Memorial Hospital. I met Harvard, and my private practice was blooming just two blocks from the beach. For years, I thought that the ocean was probably good for human health; but why? Was this a myth, or was something really happening? One night in 2003, I started a preliminary research project trying to gather information about the medical uses of ocean water. Again, the mystery was revealed…I couldn't find anything about seawater medical uses at home or in hospitals. Even better, just a few articles were published in prestigious medical journals in the United States and Europe that mentioned the uses of "simple" sea baths to treat medical conditions. I couldn't believe it, and I requested a professional research at the local university medical library. I tried to buy at least a bottle of ocean water, but no pharmacy or beauty company carried such an item in the United States during that winter.

The result was very similar to the experienced university librarians. At that moment, my idea was born to learn the benefits that ocean water had on the human body. I thought I could attempt to explain the implications and the applications of seawater effectively to reconnect humans to the ocean. I thought of the multiple uses it could have. I saw images in my mind about the micro algae fighting bacteria and fungi in the lungs. I called it "the antibiotic wars"; a natural competition of the micro-elements and humans getting all the benefits. The connection has been unfortunately missed in the evolution of medicine. I thought that this might be my scientific assignment and a very personal breakthrough in life. A sunset in the town of Surfside, Florida, marked the beginning. I started by asking permission to the deities of the sea—and they were happy.

I was conflicted at the beginning of my research with the unfortunate perception by many people that seawater is harsh on the skin. That concept is wrong. Of course, it can be harsh if you stay on the beach all day exposed to the intense sun, dry sand and the silent dehydration that usually accompanies such an adventure on the seashores. Equally aggressive could be a day by the river, the lake, or in the snow. The sea is not only innocuous, but it's prudently necessary for a healthy skin. In adequate amounts and careful exposure to its chemistry, the ocean might be an unpaired source of fun and health.

SeaMyst Corporation was the result and the instrument to execute the beautiful projects involving medical uses of solutions originating with ocean water. Our vision is beyond what we have already discovered and created. It's our goal to help protect the living seas, the ocean eco systems and to help create a conscience about the radical importance of the seas for our existence as humans.

A complete chapter is dedicated to describing the new breakthroughs in the development of ***Sea~Mar***® as well as a brief description of centers around the world that are dedicated to marine therapy. History is touched, a patent is reviewed, a scientific article is reprinted with all its original contents, and new secrets are revealed for future applications of ocean water or solutions that were started from its matrix.

I hope this book can bring clear messages to the reader. From the concrete scientific findings about how the ocean helps the human body, to a greater appreciation of the sea that is already a literal part of our blood. *Marine Therapy* is not a dream or a distant hope anymore. It's a reality, and as an editorial team, we are proud because "we bring the ocean to you."

Jose A. Soto, M.D., author

2..."And the spirit of God moved upon the face of the waters.

6 And God said, Let there be a firmament in the midst of the waters, and let it divide the waters from the waters.

10...And the gathering together of the waters called He Seas: and God saw that it was good.

20 And God said, Let the waters bring forth abundantly the moving creature that hath life...

21 And God created great whales, and every living creature that moveth, which the waters brought forth abundantly, after their kind, and every winged fowl after his kind: and God saw that it was good".

The Old Testament.The First Book of Moses, called **Genesis**. Chapter 1. The Bible.

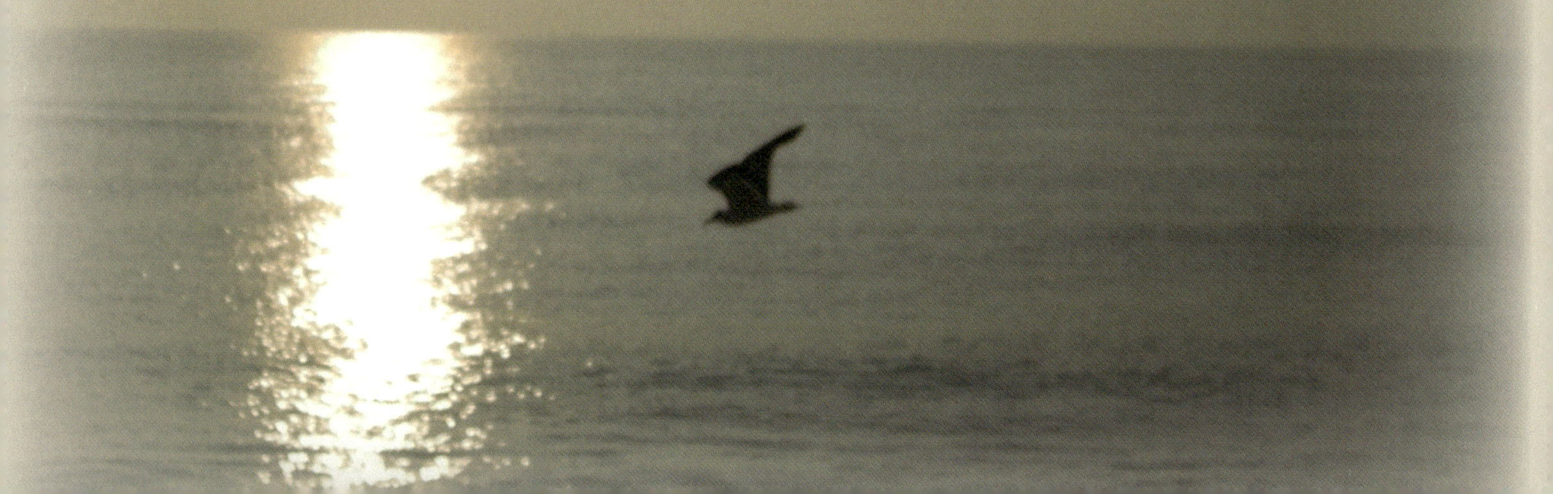

In the beginning...

The ocean is the amniotic fluid of mankind. Standing in front of the ocean is like standing in front of our whole life as a species. The sea is probably as old as the planet Earth itself. The ocean chemistry suffered dramatic changes with the earlier volcanic activity, cataclysms, and the glacial periods; however, according to recent publications, the sea chemistry has probably remained the same for millions of years. The last mass extinction of species occurred approximately sixty-five million years ago.

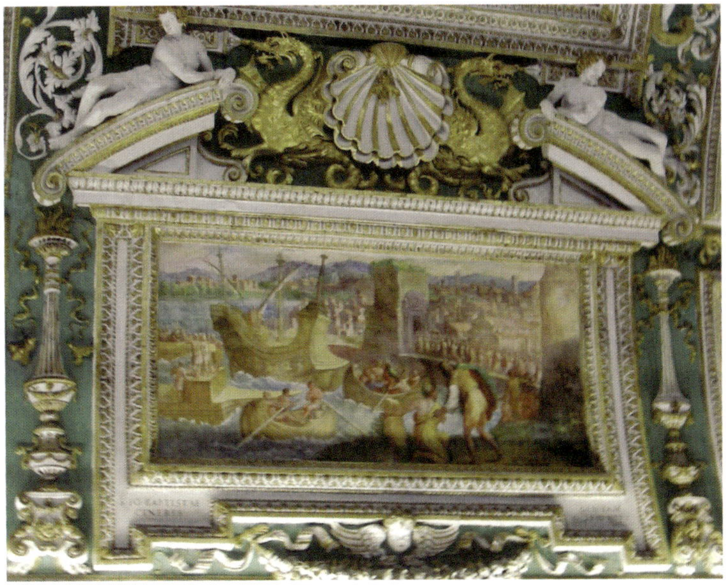

This was the last era of the dinosaurs and the marine reptiles. Definitely a change in the sea's chemistry could have been a result or a consequence of this massive loss.

Proto Indian cultures from the Harappan civilization created what is believed today as the first tidal dock, around 2300 B.C. on the coast of Gujarat, India. There are multiple citations found on the Internet about Hippocrates (460-355 B.C.) and references to the therapeutic uses of seawater, especially in his famous *Treaty of Medicine*, where the so-called Father of Modern Medicine described the uses of seawater for healing the hands of the fishermen. **Thalassotherapy** is also a word of Greek origins created to designate the uses of seawater with healing purposes. The Romans added to the concept of using seawater for more than a transportation environment to navigate between territories. They adored the ocean and saw it as a source of life. Neptune was for the Romans what Poseidon was for the Greeks—the goddess of the seas. However, it wasn't just a simple copy, but goddesses of autochthones origins on each civilization. The influence of the Roman appreciation of the ocean is still visible. Ruins in Pompeii despite mosaics in the *Terme Stabbina* (79 B.C.) with maritime motives, very especially, a child riding a dolphin, were considered a symbol of good luck.

There is a beautifully preserved mosaic floor at the *Terme di Nettuno* (Neptune thermal) in the *Ostia Antica* (the Old Roman Port).

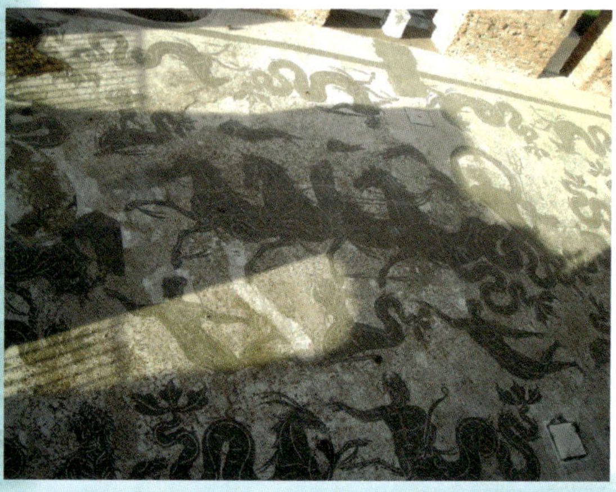

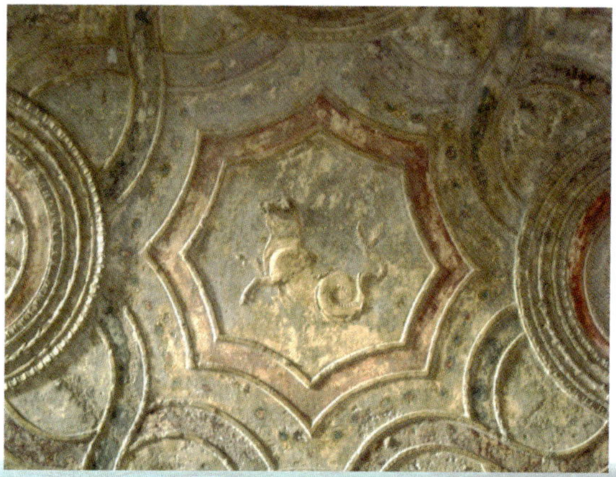

Neptune is clearly recognized on his solid shell chariot pulled by a *quadriga* of four sea horses riding in a brave sea.

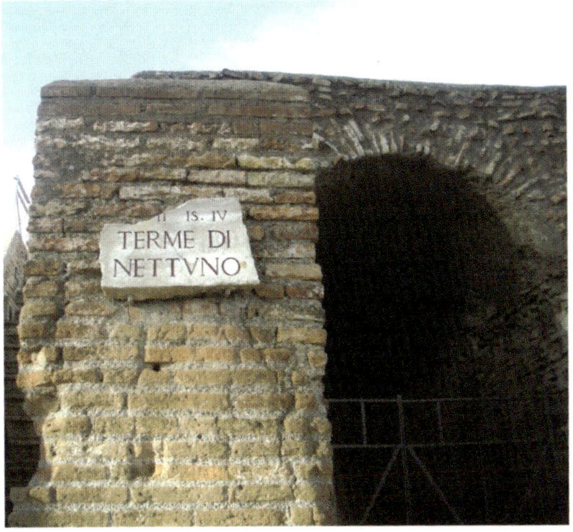

The Romans recognized the effects of water on the skin by applying methods that used hot water, warm water, and cold water on the skin for health purposes *(caldarium, tepidarium and frigidarium)*. They also used open pools *(natatio)* that were located in the open air, steaming rooms (saunas) and smaller pools similar to the Jacuzzi of today.

Big pools or smaller baths similar to the Jacuzzi of today, were used indistinctively. Notice the detail on the base of the column located in the Thermal of Neptune in the Ostia Antica, the old Roman port close to the capital. The base of the column appears to be of a coral origin. If proven real, it wouldn't be unrealistic to think about the possible uses of seawater for cosmetic and healing purposes. The detail reveals a significant difference from the surrounding structures made of brick, marble, and stucco. It's said that in the old Babylon, physicians were called *A-Su*, meaning "one who knows water." The reverence is visible everywhere and much more has been recorded in religious passages.

The Sea, the God, and the Human

The word **ocean,** or to be more precise, *Oceanus,* comes from the Greek *Okeanos.* It originated to name the god of all the salty waters. The ocean was considered in antiquity as a massive river that ran around the world. Later, Oceanus was mostly accepted as the god for what is known today as the Atlantic Ocean and Poseidon later, as some scholars believe, was the god of the Mediterranean Sea.

The sea, as a natural wonder, has been a source of existential meditations for centuries. Philosophers, historians, artists, scientists, explorers, politicians, doctors, chemists, and definitely sailors of all kinds, have found on the sea a reason for their deepest thoughts. There is a link between the power of the seas, the magic of the sound, the essence of life, and the very existence of the man and God. The sea has been perceived as a god that deserves respect, tributes, and a permanent place in our short existence in life. The Vikings were convinced of this fact, but they also found its practical value as the way to survive beyond their known world. Other cultures had the same perceptions, but only these days all this information can be compiled in a sea of megabytes.

Yemayá

The sea has been a source of inspiration and practical uses since the pre-Christian era. It has been documented that the Yoruba religion in Africa (originated in approximately 400 B.C.) venerated *Yemayá* as the goddess of the seas. Religious beliefs were brought to America by the African slaves and the cultural phenomena survived miraculously, mostly in Cuba, but also in Brazil, Haiti and other countries. *Yemayá* is represented in Afro-Caribbean rituals as an *Oricha* (a goddess) dressed in blue and white. She is considered the ocean itself, and the mother divinity who can cure infertility. She is considered the original matter and her children are the living things in the ocean. It has been recorded that she blesses everything related to the seas, including healing processes, procreation, spiritual cleansing, and the blessing from a goddess closer to *Olofi*—the Almighty God.

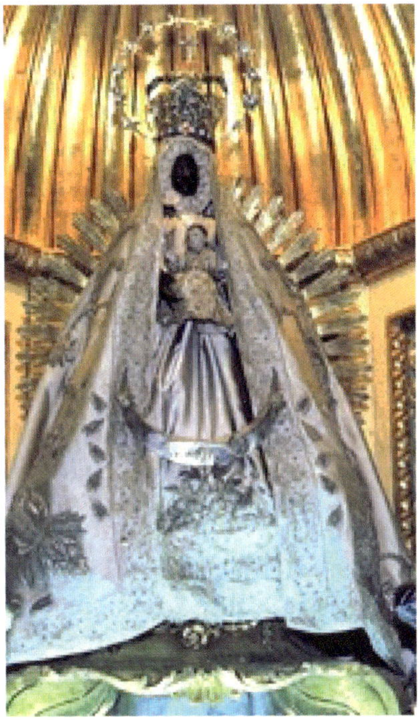

Yemayá is a deity or *Oricha* in the Afro-Cuban *Santería* religion. Syncretized, she is represented as *Nuestra Señora la Virgen de Regla*. In Brazil, she is named *YemanjÃi* or *lemanjÃi,* and in Haiti, she is *La SirÃ¨ne* (The Mermaid in the Vodou religion). She is the mother sea. She is identified with the number seven or any combination of seven—a clear connection to the traditional seven seas. Her colors are blue and white. Offerings to *Yemayá* include seven coins, blue and white candles, salt, salt water, boats, shellfish, shells and seaweed. She is the nurturer of all. She can show her temper or be peaceful. *Yemayá* is *Ochun's* sister, *Oricha* of the rivers.

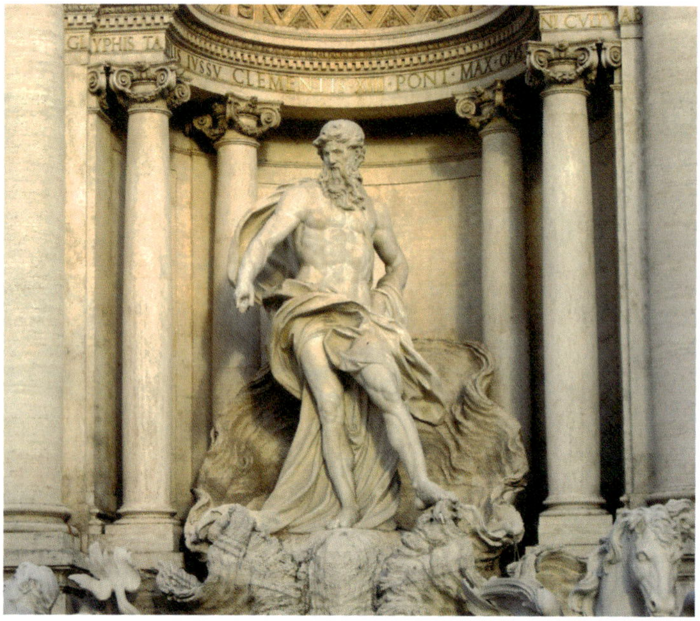

Neptune

In Roman mythology, there is only space for one deity to rule the seas. *Neptune* was a horse deity of Etruscan origins. He is depicted sometimes as an old man, bearded, wise, strong, and scary when furious. *Neptune* always carries a trident. He is bearded and seen in association with dolphins and fish. One of his children was *Triton*. *Neptune's* powers were documented in the Homeric *Aeneid* where he saved Trojan sailors.

Poseidon

Poseidon was a Greek deity venerated in the Olympus as brother of *Zeus* and considered a lord of the seas. He is represented with a trident that he can also use to shake the Earth with his powers. Sometimes he's represented as a warrior on a shell carriage pulled by horses. The Greeks were considered an awesome force in the Mediterranean Sea. The veneration of *Poseidon* was recorded in *The Iliad.* Both *Poseidon* and *Neptune* were equivalent representations of the same divinity in each mythology—the Greek and the Roman. Both were gods of the same vast sea and of the humans that even today put their trust in them.

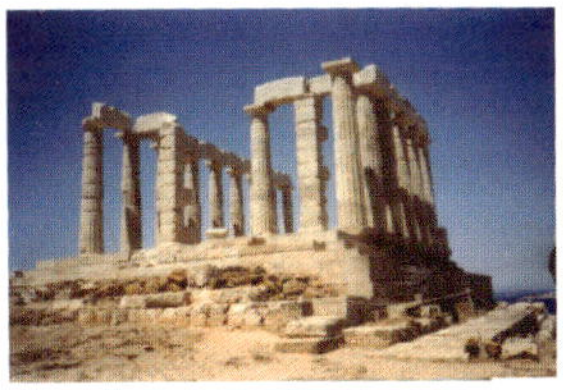

The Conservatory Museum in Rome has preserved the *Dea Roma* (Roma Goddess) from the times of Caesar in the antiquity. A maritime symbol in the form of a seashell is depicted over the throne of the goddess in her majestic image.

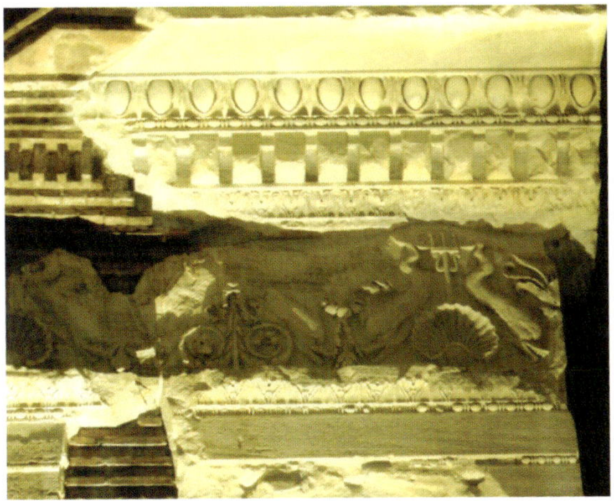

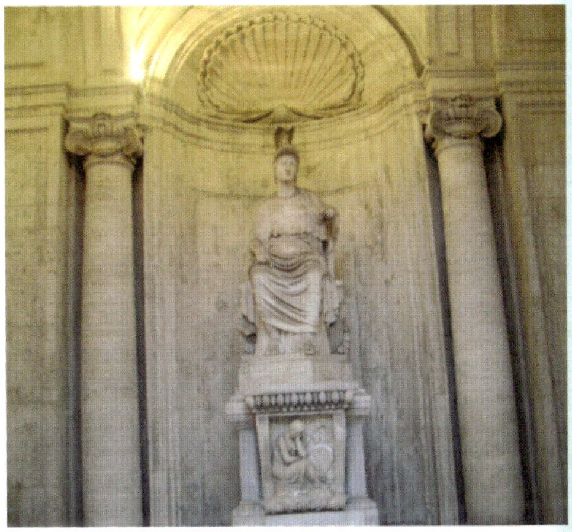

Right behind the Roman Pantheon there is a *petite* street where you can appreciate the meticulous work that appears over the top of the columns. Decorating the posterior façade with maritime elements are a trident, fishes (or dolphins) and shells that form a decorative pattern. This attention to detail confirms that early Italians were fascinated by the sea; just 2,000 years ago.

Leonardo da Vinci

Leonardo da Vinci made studies about water. He dedicated time to analyze the patterns of water motion and turbulence as depicted on his *Sheets of Study of Water* treasured at the Windsor Castle Royal Library. Leonardo, as a great observer, noticed the intrinsic force of the liquid and its potentials to generate energy that could be preserved and transported long distances through canals.

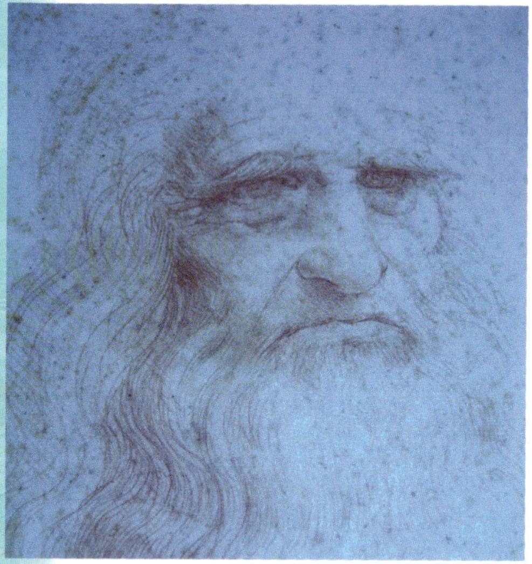

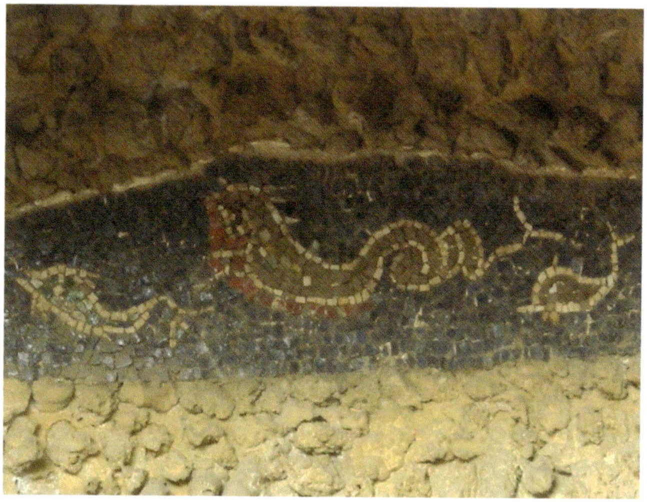

He compared the motion of water with the motion of hair. His drawings show the turbulent effects of streams passing different obstacles. On his paintings, Leonardo da Vinci frequently used water views of lakes, rivers, or "the oceanic sea" as he graciously called it. The great painter used the sea views mostly as a decorative element for the background. There is no doubt in my mind that Leonardo could be a great marine life researcher considering his extraordinary observation capacity, drawing skills, talent for classification, and the genius to develop methods and instruments

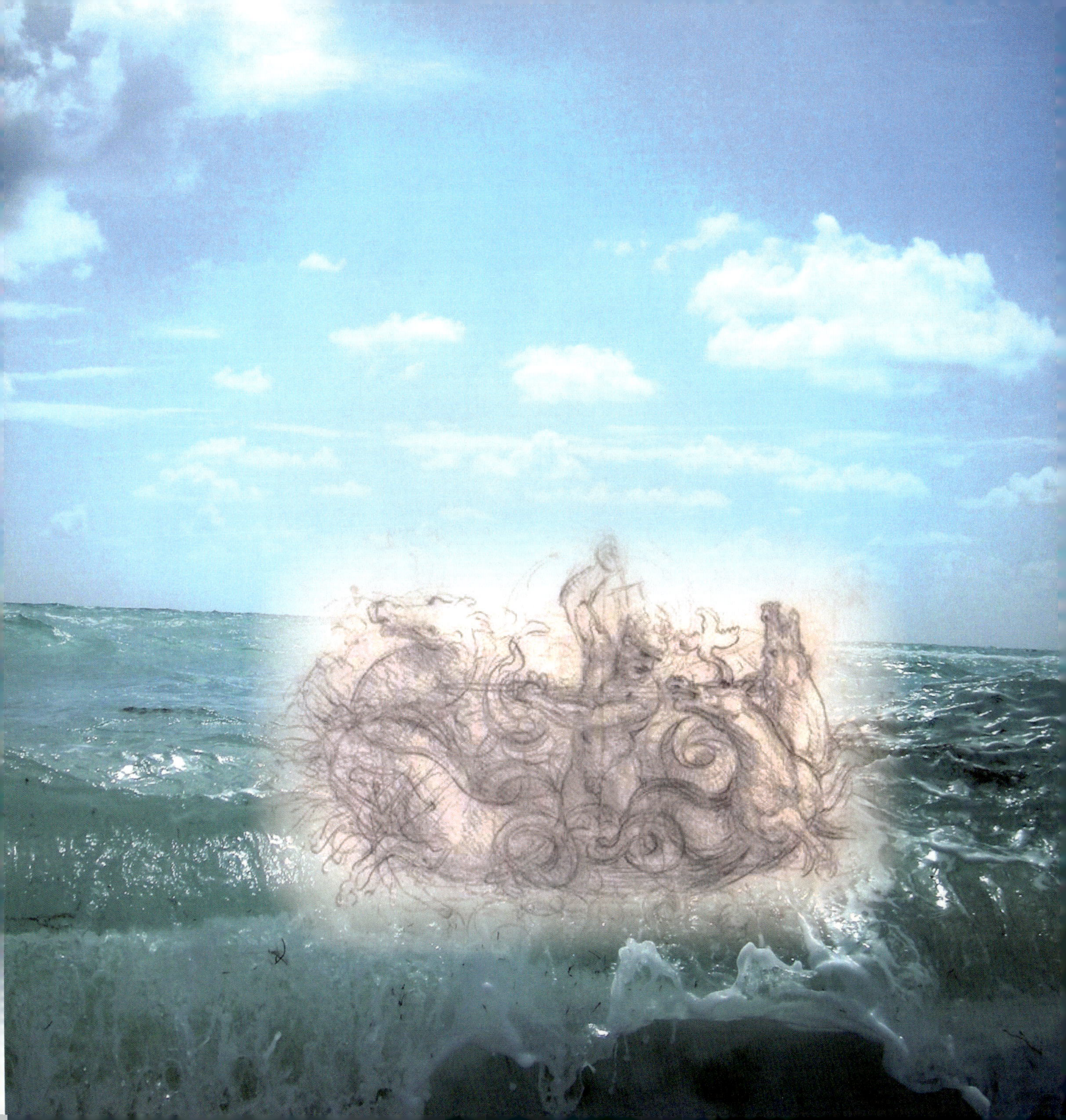

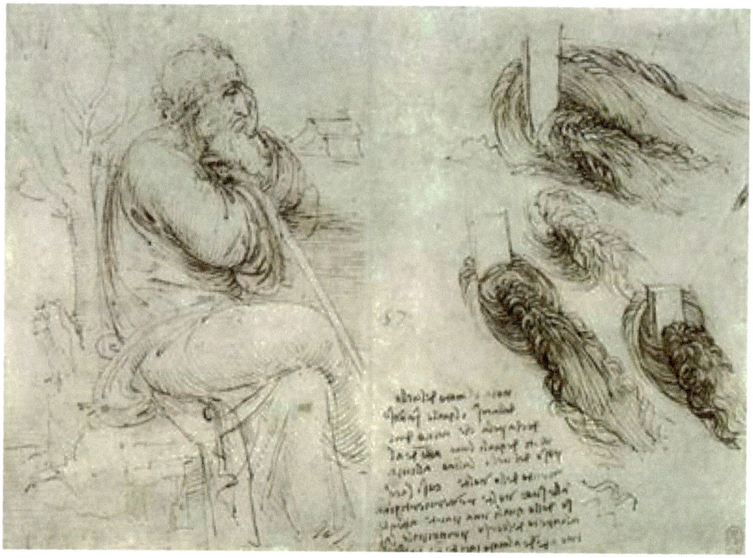

In the Renaissance monuments, paintings and fountains made numerous mentions of the sea and sea-related elements. From the Vatican galleries to the popular streets of modern capitals, the ocean has fascinated engineers, painters, and sculptors of many generations.

The maps gallery in the Vatican Museum is rich in the ocean representations. In this particular painting, the frame and the painting clearly represent the importance of the sea in human life.

The *Fontana di Trevi* in the *Cittá d' Acqua* in Rome was built by the architect Salve in the times of Clement XIII. The man standing represents the ocean (or Neptune by others) and he is surrounded by marine elements including seahorses, Titans, shells, snails, corals, and plants.

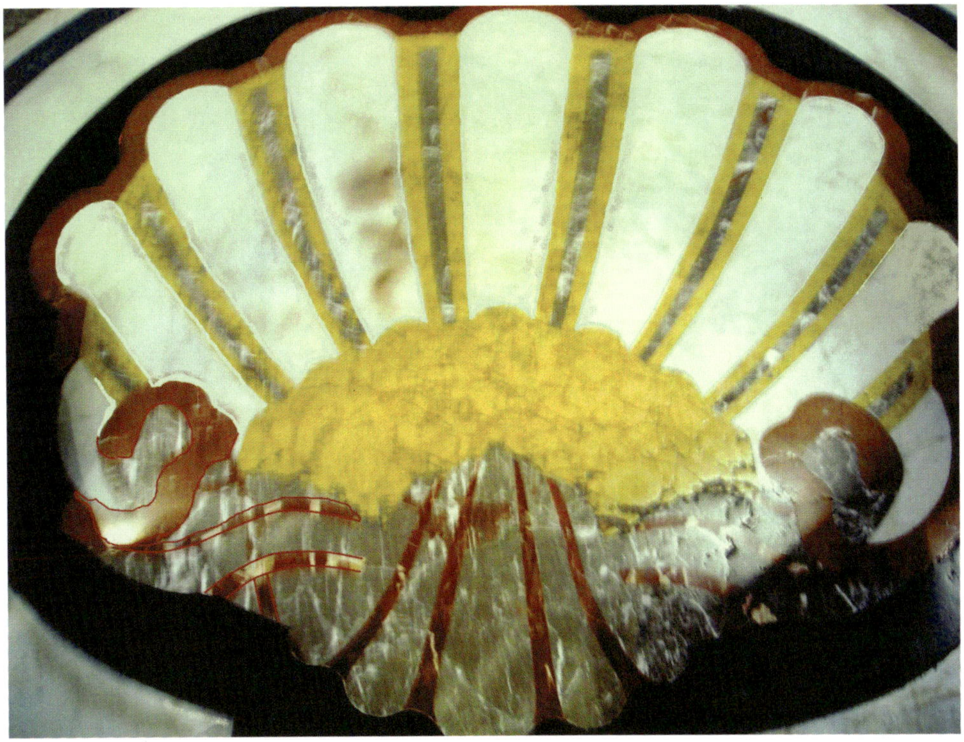

Seashell-shaped mosaic at the Saint Peter's Church floor in Vatican City, Italy.

The king and queen of France were called the *Dauphin* and the *Dauphiné* (which is the French word for "dolphin"). This was clearly related to the fact that the Coat of Arms had two magnificent marine animals and mammals, which were considered part of the evolutionary theory—the dolphins.

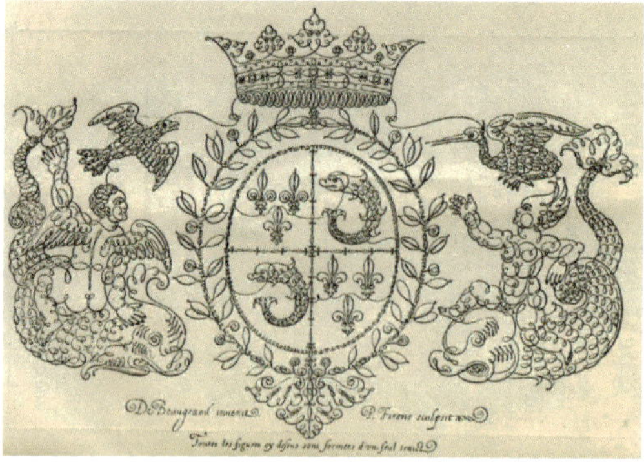

The Coat of Arms was created by Jean de Beaugrand in 1604, but the dolphin was also present in the Vienne Coat of Arms.

Alexander Marcet

Dr. Alexander John Gaspar Marcet (1770-1822) was a physician and chemist from Switzerland, who discovered the sea's key element's composition in the nineteenth century. Dr. Marcet studied seawater samples from different parts of the world. He noticed that there was a variation in the contents of salt in the water of different areas. He discovered in 1819 that the proportions of the major constituents of seawater never changed, even when the salinity of the water did. The fact was verified later by George Forchhammer in 1865. Two years later, in 1867, Doctor de la Bonnardiere invented the word ***thalassotherapy*** from the Greek words *thallasso* (sea) and *therapy* (treatment). In 1884, William Dittmar established the "law" of constant proportions in seawater. The principle establishes that for certain amounts of the ion, chloride, there will be a proportional amount of sodium, sulfate and magnesium, even when the concentration of salt in the seawater varies.

Renee Quinton

Renee Quinton (1867-1925) was a man recognized for the leaps he achieved in ocean water analysis and applications.

Mr. Quinton was in fact a biologist and the first to propose the cell evolution from the ocean. He published his book, *Ocean, the Organic Environment* in 1904, as a way to communicate his findings and the ideas of what was later called the "Quinton's Plasma." He established that seawater was indeed a live habitat, and had an atmosphere on its own. He described the organic identity existing between the seawater and the blood plasma. Mr. Quinton created a method to process seawater. He mixed it with fresh distilled water and used it as an intravascular infusion to replace blood loss or lack of nutrients in the human body. The climax was achieved when clinical experiments were performed using the application of Quinton's plasma through the mammal's circulatory system.

In France, at the beginning of the twentieth century, Quinton's plasma was used in animals with seawater as plasma for intravascular administration. The animals (dogs) survived the experience. The scandal brought to light that the components of the ocean were very similar to those in the human serum. In 1906, he opened the first marine dispensary in Paris. It's said that French soldiers received Quinton's plasma infusion after the blood supplies were depleted during the First World War. "Quinton's Plasma" was the name given to the process that used the ocean water in animals and eventually in humans; particularly in undernourished children, patients with psoriasis, eczema and other problems documented with pictures by physicians of that era.

Alexander Oparin (1894-1980), a renowned Russian scientist, formulated his theory about the sea acting as the primary source of life in the planet. In 1924, he explained to the world that intense radiation acting over the elements present in the ocean could generate simple chemical structures that might later evolve into more complex forms of life, like the cell.

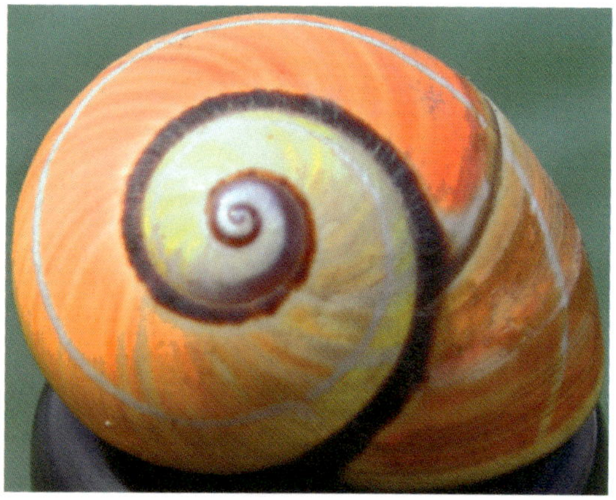

Oparin's theory was backed up by extraordinary experiments.

The Seawater and Its Properties

Seawater is the critical portion of the ocean that allows everything else to prosper and where all living matter exists. It's almost magical. It exists and persists no matter what. It's much more than salt and water; actually, it's not that simple. **Seawater is a compound**—a perfect mix of elements **in constant proportions**. Do you want me to complicate this more? Those elements are electrically charged (they are called ions), and they're responsible for the salty taste of seawater. The ions are completely dissolved and I have found evidence that they remain and interact with each other and with the living matters, including our bodies.

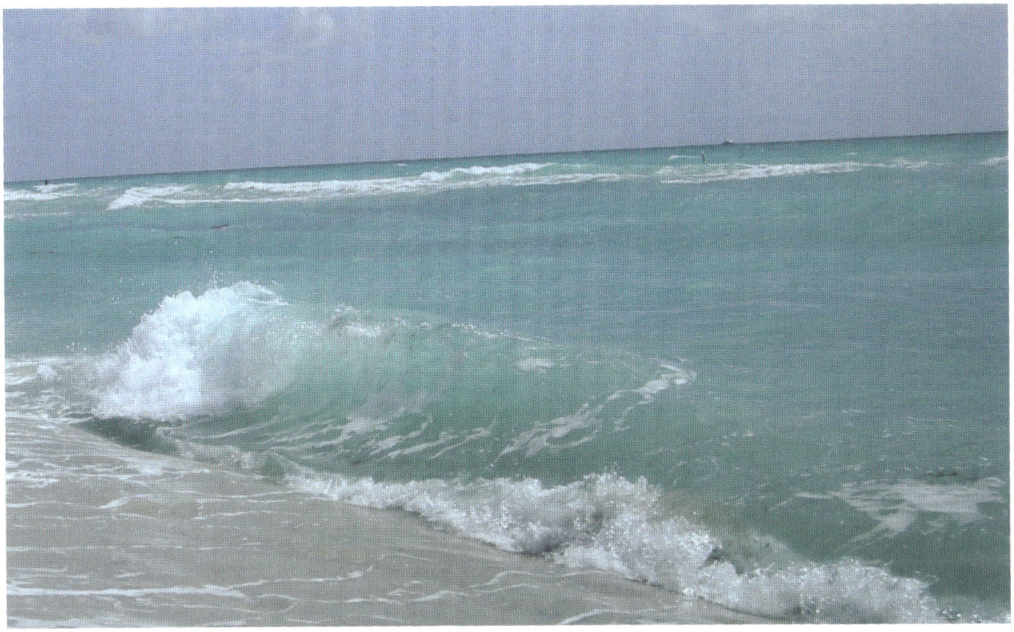

Although there are **more than eighty natural chemical elements in the ocean,** some ions are considered "key" due to their proportion and quantities. Ocean water is actually a huge jungle of living elements, all the biggest animals of the kingdom, and the smallest, as well. Everything is important for something else that at the same time is critical for other reactions or organisms. It's a chain of events that happens every second of our existence—even before and after, for millions of years.

When I started separating the beach water from all the elements present in it, I ended up with a chemical solution. I saw that it looked like glass—clear, transparent and powerful. After sending samples to the laboratory, I found that the solution was composed of the classical **six key elements—sodium, potassium, calcium, magnesium, chloride, and sulfate.** Those are the most abundant and they are also the most common and critical ions in our human blood. That's not a coincidence. We have an ocean *DNA*. This is probably the strongest genetic and chemical evidence that we have evolved from the sea, or not?

The ions are dissolved in H20 (water) and they are active. I have found that they form compounds that dissolve back into their natural state or they continue interacting to form other compounds, Again, it's an endless cycle of energy that opens the doors for numerous applications. The fact that these ions are electrically charged allows them to interact with our cells as proven in the pictures taken and described later in this book. This is the case—the cells are formed by membranes and organelles, which are the little internal organs of the cell body. The membranes are the walls, but those walls are highly selective in the way they allow substances to penetrate our body. The cell membranes use ions like messengers to interact with the environment. These ions are exactly like those that are found in the ocean. The most important cellular ions found in the human body are sodium, potassium, chloride, magnesium, and calcium. Is this a coincidence? Of course, it is not. More than that, it's definitely evidence of a connection. Have you ever tasted your sweat, or your own tears? The main components—sodium and chloride are the most common elements in seawater. We are the ocean.

The Physical Properties

Seawater is mostly liquid, but it might be found on earth frozen and even in the form of gas sprayed over the coast or the ships when the seas are roughed by the wind and the currents. Seawater is also very compact in structure. It's heavier than fresh water. Water has been wisely called the universal solvent. **It dissolves practically everything,** so ocean water is possibly **the best vehicle to transport any other chemical or biological element** that needs to be absorbed into the human body.

The atoms are so tight that if you fall on the water from a third floor building, it might be like falling on cement. This property is called **high surface tension**. The energy produced by a wave can be so destructive that gigantic manmade structures like buildings and seawalls can be destroyed in a blink of time by the impact of the waves.

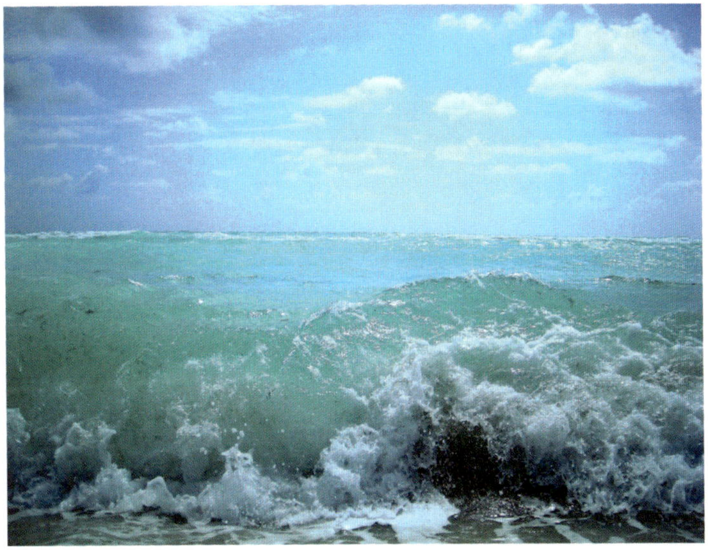

Water is composed of two elements—oxygen and hydrogen. Two *cations* (which are ions charged positively) bond with one anion, oxygen, which is charged negatively. The union is created through bonds that are very flexible, and which allow a change to occur in the shape of the molecules when they aggregate. The molecules of H2O are very tight. This high surface tension is also important for the interaction with the skin and organs such as the lungs, as proven later on.

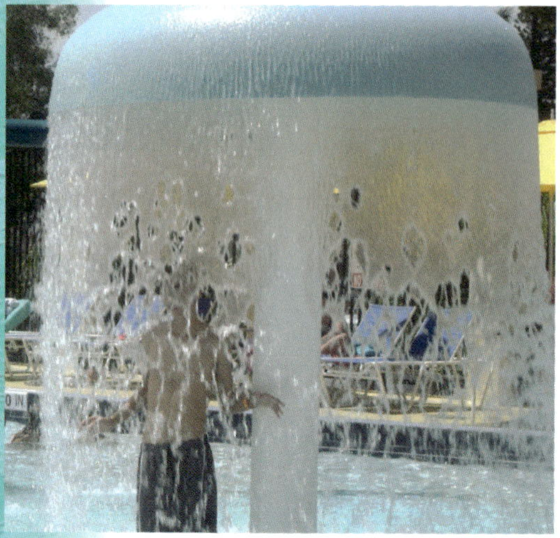

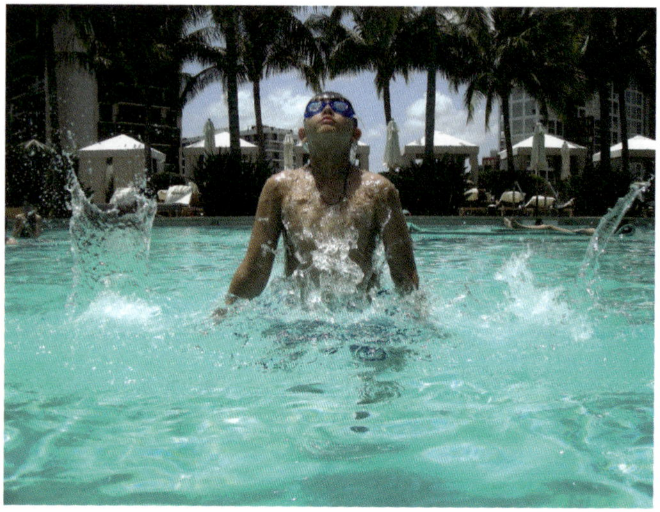

The water's **high surface tension** also allows the formation of interesting phenomena like rivers, streams, currents, waterfalls, whirlpools, waves, or simple drops of water. Big barrel-shaped waves are formed thanks to the tension that results from the interaction between the molecules of oxygen and hydrogen. As mentioned above, ocean water also has other ionic elements that add more surface tension to the precious liquid. This strong tension between the elements allows not only a tight formation of drops over the skin or other surfaces, but the floating of huge vessels made of cement and steel. Strong surface tension may allow the flotation of objects not made to float, like a simple paper clip. Scientific experiments have proved that purified ocean water has a direct effect over other liquids, like human secretions from the respiratory tract.

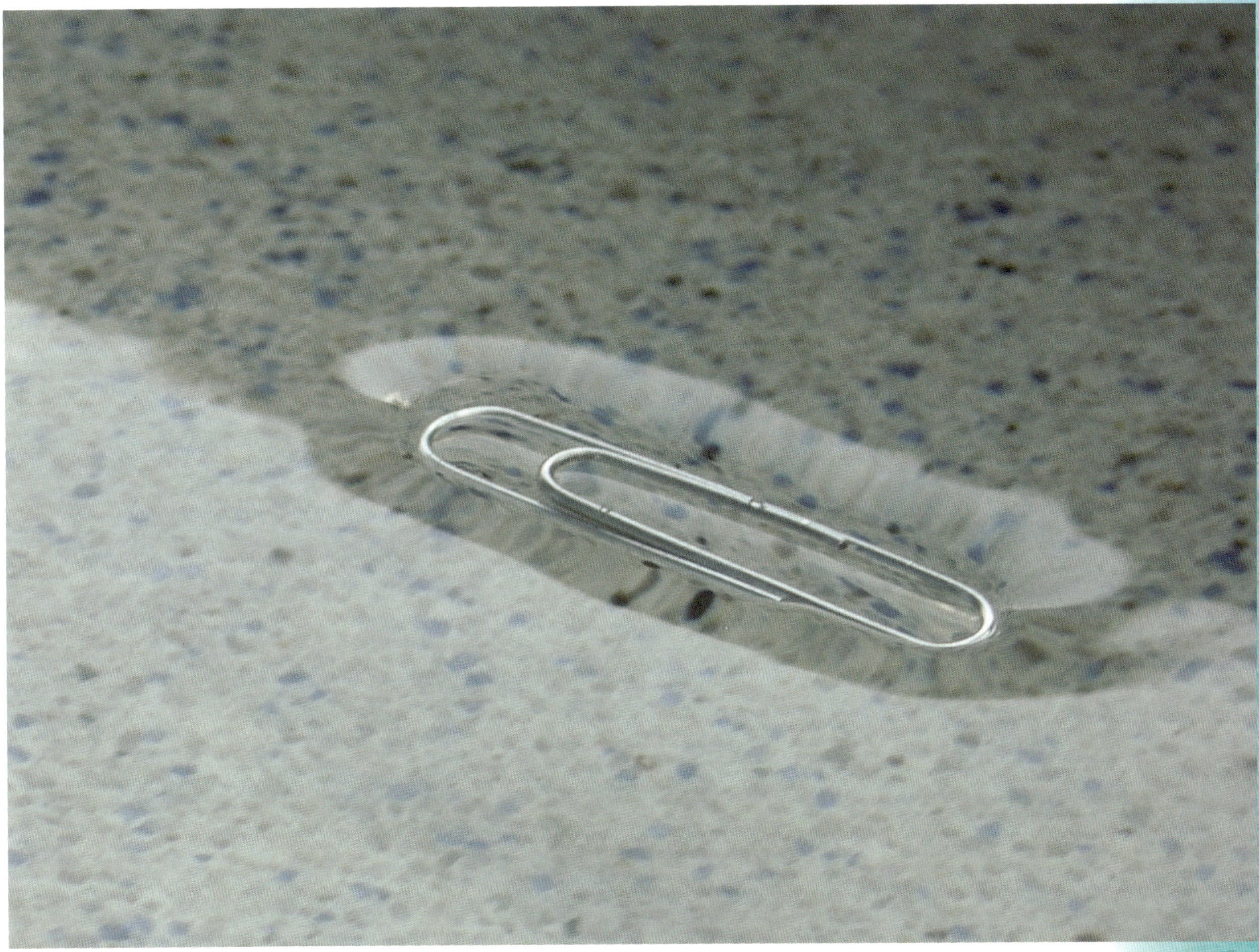

The close interaction between the two hydrogen molecules and the oxygen allows the water to act as a solid structure that holds a piece of metal floating like a leaf. This property not only allows navigation, but it could allow the ocean water to be used in aerosols for medical treatments.

When we combine the properties of the water and the chemical advantages of the key elements present in the ocean, we have an extraordinary substance—the compound of compounds; a unique matter in the known universe that might cautiously be considered the original matter of Earth life. Water can be frozen, or in the form of micro particles, it can be suspended in the air and called an aerosol or simply a vapor.

Seawater has another property that is just as amazing—its **high refreshing capacity or heat absorption**. Seawater is more refreshing on the skin than alcohol or acetone. Different from these substances, seawater doesn't leave the skin dry. Actually, the skin becomes softer and smoother. It's incredibly more refreshing than the gas used in any refrigerator or air-conditioning system, such as Freon 12. This property makes the ocean a natural anti-inflammatory; probably the best. Seawater might absorb all the heat in an area (earth or animal body) thanks to its natural composition. So, let's say theoretically, that if an area is swollen, it's surely warm, red and likely *edematous* (swollen). If seawater is placed in contact with that area, it will probably refresh, causing cooling and vasoconstriction (a phenomena related to a decrease in redness and possibly edema). In addition to that, the ions present in the ocean water will interact with the area. It will penetrate the cells and activate mechanisms to promote an electrical exchange. This is more than figurative. The pictures disclosed in the next chapter confirm the scientific theories. Clinical studies need to be done to confirm this amazing discovery.

Alchemy of God

Seawater is a very stable chemical compound. In my laboratory, for more than four years, I have stored closed bottles of the solution that was started from ocean water; stored at the environmental temperature in South Florida. The elements remain active and they change their quantities as expected in a chemical reaction that never stops taking place; however, the solution remains stable. Why doesn't it decompose?

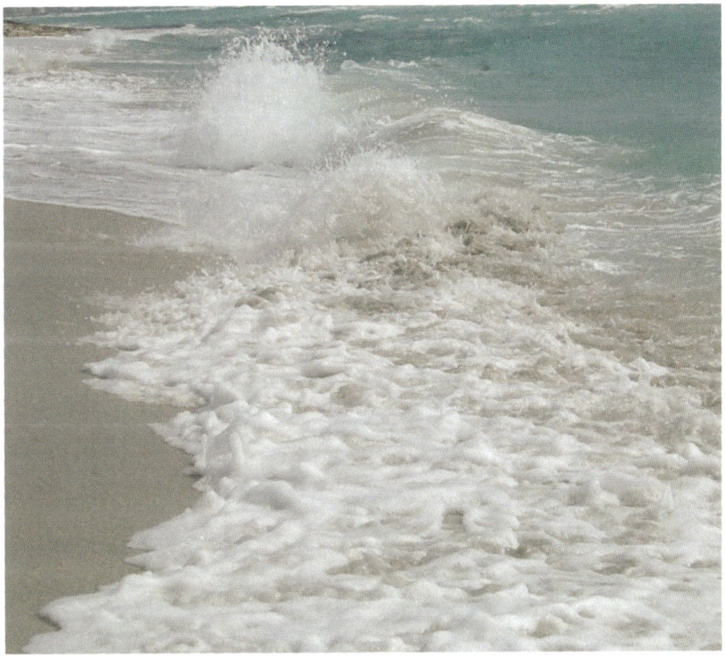

I have observed something quite interesting. The answer probably is that **the sea ions have a unique distribution and arrangement in the periodic table of natural elements**. I have found that the key elements are positioned in the table almost in a sequential way from the positions eleventh to twentieth. More than that, the elements are located in pairs as follows: Sodium (Na)

and Magnesium (Mg) in the eleventh and twelfth positions; Sulfate (S) and Chloride (Cl) in the sixteenth and seventeenth positions; and Potassium (K) and Calcium (Ca) in the nineteenth and twentieth positions. Those charged positive Sodium (Na), Calcium (Ca), Magnesium (Mg), and Potassium (K) are associated very proximally to each other. The ones charged negatively—Chloride (Cl) and Sulfur (S) are also next to each other and occupy an intermediate position on the table. I believe this provides the compound with an extraordinary stability because each element has very similar chemical properties to the next one. Also as a group of elements, they are aligned in almost a continuous sequence; something that I have never heard of in any natural substance or compound. That is why the bottles with purified ocean water treated by our method might have such a prolonged shelf life. This is a very important aspect in commerce. More than eighty elements have been discovered in ocean water ***(Handbook of Chemistry and Physics,*** 65th Ed. 1984-85, CRC Press, Boca Raton, Florida p. F-149)

This is probably why the ocean has remained as is for millions of years. To the ocean, it doesn't matter if there's radiation or rain, cold or hot weather, storms or earthquakes. The ocean water always remains stable and we are all responsible for the protection of this stability.

Practical Applications

I. Skin

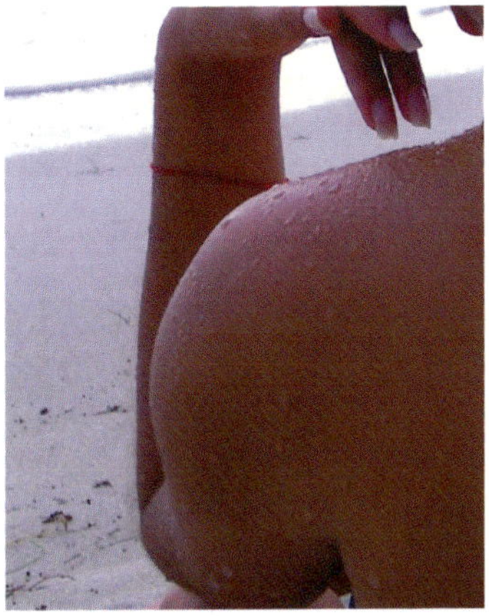

Ocean water and sea salts have an extraordinary impact in the human body. The following is a compilation of information extracted from scientific articles published by prestigious medical journals. I have written the key phrases and have added a short explanation of the significance of the findings. They refer to the uses of solutions containing salt or simply seawater, for the treatment of medical problems or just due to their cosmetic effects. The investigative reports have been used as the scientific background for our commitment to bring the ocean to the public. The analysis from the author and the scientific quotes are followed by a bibliographic citation of the article.

The conclusions of the scientist can't be bolder—"bathing in water with a high salt concentration, including the ocean water is safe, effective, and pleasant for healing and recovery. This approach needs no chemicals or potentially harmful drugs." There are almost no side effects during and after the treatment, and there is a very low risk to the patient's general well-being." (*Matz, Orion, and Wolf in "Balneotherapy in Dermatology" (**Dermatology Therapy**, vol. 16, page 132, June 2003*).)

Effects on the Immune System

Japanese scientists have recently published the impressive effects of Deep Sea Water (DSW) in the human immune system.

The study is a pioneer work involving the uses of marine water extracted from depths beyond one hundred feet. The explanation is simple. The ocean water causes an anti-inflammatory effect that increases the number of cells that act to calm down or suppress allergic types of reactions.

Bathing in hot deep seawater produced an increase in human lymphocytes (CD8 or suppressor type), which relates to anti-inflammatory effects; all of which may explain the observation of improvement in some skin diseases characterized by inflammation. (*Tschiya, Shimizu, Tazawa et al.*

in "Effects of Hot Deep Seawater Bathing on the Inmune Cell Distribution in Peripheral Blood from Healthy Young Men" in ***Environ. Health Prev. Med.****, Vol. 8, pp. 161-165 (2003).)*

Deep Sea Water (DSW) is also extracted near Hawaii, from "the conveyor belt," and has been used in combination with artificial elements in the cosmetic industry. DSW is collected from depths that keep the water colder, denser, and with significantly more salinity.

Cosmetic Effects

I think of the purified ocean water as the perfect cosmetic. Its benefits on the skin are beyond anything expected. First, purified ocean water is good for any skin type. It has no significant side effects. It has long lasting activity, causes no allergies, and produces a perennial smoothness.

A group of doctors decided to study the smoothing effects on the skin of the ocean water, the Mediterranean seawater, and the Dead Sea minerals. The article was published in 1997. The authors proved that "all three treatments have been proven to be significantly effective in smoothing the skin's surface." This study was done using very precise methods of skin analysis (profilometric), which reduced the margin of error on the interpretation of results. The measurements of the skin changes could be repeated by anybody who wanted to test on his own. It's just amazing what seawater can do to our nature. (*Ma'or and Voss, "Skin Smoothing Effects of Dead Sea Minerals: Comparative Profilometric Evaluation of Skin Surface." 1997.* ***International Journal of Cosmetic Science,*** *Vol. 19, Number 1.*)

Japanese scientists have studied the skin cell effects of minerals present in seawater. In a study published in 2004, they have concluded that the minerals present in ocean water can act as humectants and they may even accelerate the production of collagen by the cells called fibroblasts. So, according to this study, if you frequently go to the beach, you're probably stimulating your immune system and getting firmer and stronger skin. Collagen provides stability to the skin tissues that make then tight. Collagen is like flexible cement or natural glue. Fibroblasts are cells related to the skin's healing process and they produce collagen. *(M. Ooe, H. Okumura, T. Yamamura, H. Matsunaka, T. Morioka (2004) "Repair of Dry Skin By Minerals In Seawater: OLIGOMARINE® as a Skin Moisturizer." 2004.* ***International Journal of Cosmetic Science*** *26 (6), 316–316. doi:10.1111/j.1467-2494.)*

Effects Described in Psoriasis and Atopic Dermatitis

Psoriasis is not a simple skin disease. Not so much for the intensity of the pain, but for the presence of lesions that may scare the patients and other people. Psoriasis is not contagious—at all! Psoriasis is an inflammatory disease characterized by lesions that turn the skin red, swollen, dry, and flaky. The disease is not inherited and again, not transmissible. Atopic dermatitis is also a skin problem associated with inflammation of the skin that makes it itchy, red, and dry in selected areas of the body. Atopic dermatitis is not contagious either, but it is related to allergies in many patients.

Psoriasis and atopic dermatitis are common dermatological diseases that are frequently treated with balneotherapy with a very high success rate. Many studies published in European medical journals have described the fact that patients commonly benefit from beach baths. Is this an effect related to the relaxation than usually is associated with rest and fun by the ocean? Is there something chemical about this "magic" improvement? Of course, relaxing is beneficial for most human health problems; however, the studies reveal evidence that chemical effects are caused by the salinity of the ocean water and other sea salts like from the Dead Sea. "The combination of seawater bath and solar radiation has been proven effective in the treatment of patients affected by skin diseases such as psoriasis and dermatitis. Magnesium is the ion most likely responsible due to its activity that stimulates skin cell proliferation" (*Schemp, Dittmar, Hummler and collaborators in*

"Magnesium Ions Inhibit the Antigen-presenting function of Human Epidermal Langerhans Cells In Vivo and In Vitro. Involvement of ATPase, HLA-DR, B7 Molecules, and Cytokines" published in the **Journal of Investigative Dermatology** (2000) 115, 680-686.

If magnesium favors skin cell proliferation, it might also be responsible for the unequivocal **tanning effect of the ocean water**. Magnesium is also a chemical messenger for the cells and it may well stimulate the production of *melanine*, the skin coloring substance.

The sole visit to the beach may improve psoriatic lesions; however, bathing in a solution of sea salts and the application of a phototherapy equivalent to sun ray exposure was evaluated in a multicenter trial showing significant improvement and patient acceptance. Another study showed that natural sunlight combined with salt water bathing cleared psoriasis. ***British Journal of Dermatology,*** 1998; 139: (1012-1019).

"Trips to the beach or salt water in the bathtub followed by sunbathing can be a pleasant addition to psoriasis therapy" (**drgreen.com** accessed in 2006). In Japan, "it is empirically known that seawater is effective for the treatment of atopic dermatitis." Mechanisms by which this happens probably involve immunomodulatory, mechanical, chemical, and thermal effects. These mechanisms are not fully understood, but published results confirmed that symptoms such as pruritus can be significantly decreased after the use of sprayed purified seawater. (*Nomura, 1995 cited by Nakasone and Akeda in "The Application of Deep Seawater in Japan,"* National Research Institute of Fisheries Engineering.)

The key for future treatments of patients with these problems will probably include a combination of traditional medicine and modern pharmacological compounds. This concept may even pull the next one, which is using chemical compounds like steroids mixed with ocean water. I have mixed different medications with ocean water and there are no physical changes visible in the new compounds—no crystals, and no sedimentation; just a great mix. We will have to wait for the developments in the pharmaceutical industry.

The following pictures show a patient affected by urticaria, a problem characterized by skin irritation and wheals surrounded by *erythema* (redness). The problem is not a life-threatening situation, but sometimes causes enough discomfort and itching that it may interfere with daily routines. The sequence also showed the *before* and *after* effects of the application of a solution made of purified ocean water. The findings were published by ***The International Journal of Applied Sciences (SOFW Journal)****. Vol 134, No. 4, 2008. J. A. Soto:'Purified Ocean Water as a Cosmetic and a Therapeutic Solution').*

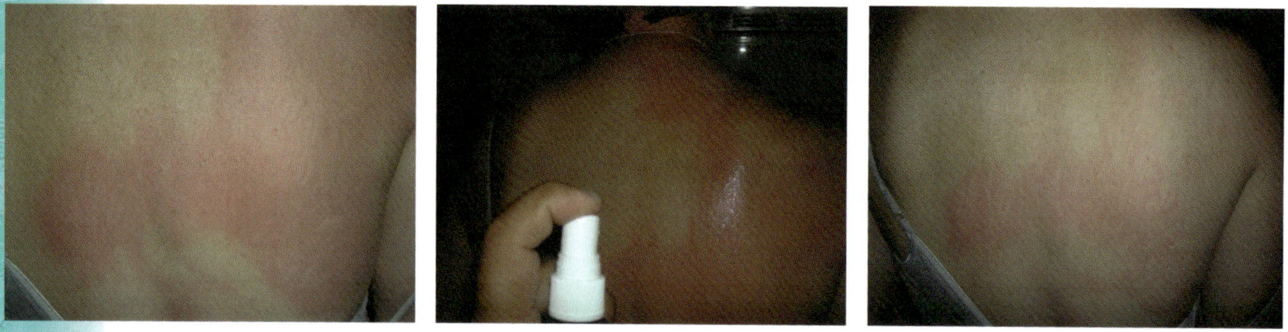

Effects of a Low Salt Solution in Acne

Also as a concomitant therapy, "water with low minerals appear to be a promising adjunctive treatment for improving the tolerance of topical retinoids in acne" (Alirezai, *Vie, Humbert, et al.* ***European Journal of Dermatology****, 2000. Volume 10, number 5, 370-2*). In this article, the authors discussed the activity of the solution and that it reduced the irritant effects of the medications used for acne. Although the compound was not precisely purified ocean water, the mechanisms involved in the uses of a low salt compound, might be similar to those of seawater to remove the stratum corneous and reduce the irritation caused by chemicals present on medications.

In dermatology, exfoliation is the physical loss of skin cells. Exfoliation caused by ocean water might be related to the presence of dissolved salts and the effects of skin massage. Other expected effects are the mechanical elimination of excess oils on the skin by a non-comedogenic substance that cleans the pores. The sweat glands as well as other excretory glands might reduce the oil production by the effect of the ions contained in ocean water. The reason why is because the cells in those glands have special pores known as aquaporins that may react to the presence of seawater, reducing the excretion of oil to the skin. Another effect is the activation of anti-inflammatory mechanisms as described by Ivyn and collaborators (**www.uspto.gov**—US Patent number *6 451 352*) after the creation of Physiomer®, a form of purified seawater. None of these articles should be considered as a conclusion or recommendation to pursue medical treatment with seawater for any of the problems here described. The words of the family doctor or the dermatologist should be the main guidance in every particular case, and you should always consult your doctor if you suffer from any dermatological condition.

All the studies consulted confirmed the benefits of sea salts in natural environments, so why not take the ocean to everybody and put it right there in the cabinet, where you can reach it every day?

The answer is *Sea~Mar®*.

It took about four years to develop fully the concept in all its expressions. The idea was subjected to a very diverse judgment pool and all of those interviewed had something in common to say—seawater is good to the human body. Many provided their opinions after seeing the ocean in a bottle, listening to the concept, or reading small pamphlets or articles created to communicate the idea. The universe of opinions was diverse—children, doctors, young women, patients, artists, entrepreneurs, cosmetologists, news reporters, people from different religions, credos, and a whole spectrum in educational level. All coincided in the simplicity and the veracity of the greatness of ocean water.

Sea~Mar® is purified ocean water prepared in a very distinctive way. It contains all the same major six elements of ocean water when compared with raw seawater. As previously mentioned, these are Sodium, Potassium, Chloride, Calcium, Magnesium, and Sulfates, which remain in the form of pharmacologically active salts or ions totally dissolved in ocean water. Its method of preparation starts with raw seawater. After a purification process, it is left in its more pure state. The final compound was the object of the patent filed by the author in the United States of America back in 2003.

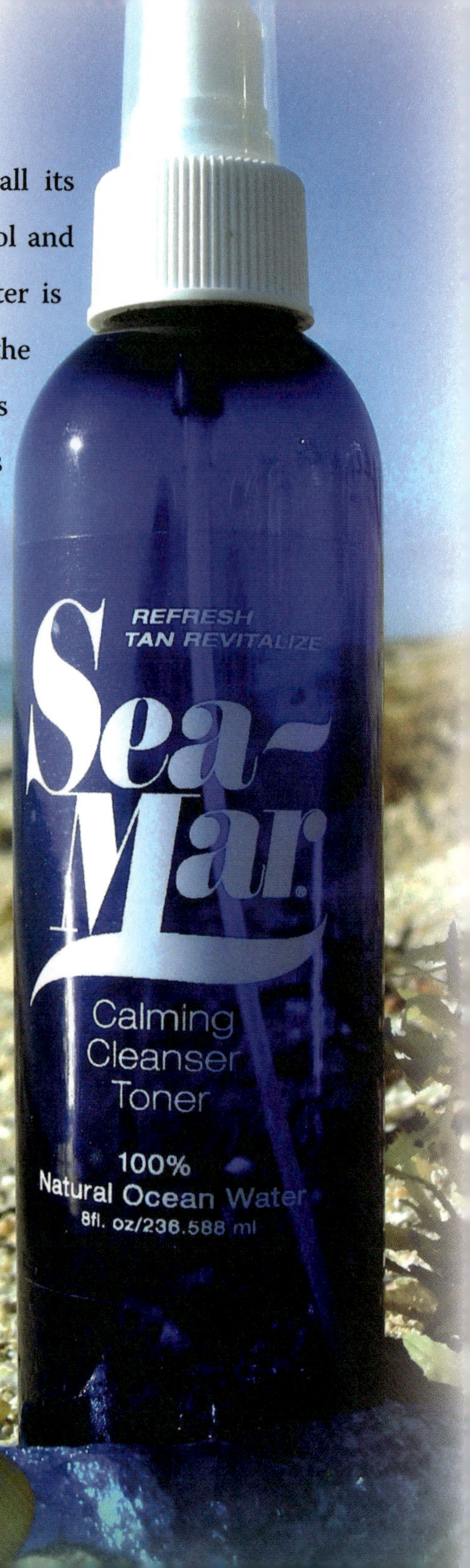

To decrease the risk of packaging undesired micro-organisms, a micro-filtration process has been perfected before the final form of distribution. A quality control system assures the product's composition and stability during the production chain. The product is much less dense than raw beach water and the natural trace elements may play a major role on the skin. Different from mud, **Sea~Mar®** is nonabrasive to the skin and easier to remove if that is desired. The active salts are in a dissolved form (ions) so the solution is always homogenous; it does not require pre-treatment shaking, since the salts remain active due to the very stable covalent bonds between the elements. They can go through a filtration process without losing their molecular properties. In other words, it is just ocean water components.

Chemical Composition

I have studied ocean water for years and I have reviewed a significant number of articles related to the main liquid in our planet. Even though it might sound obvious, I have to clarify again that seawater is not simply "table salt" dissolved in "tap water." Left to dry in the laboratory, **Sea~Mar®** forms small crystals containing different salts and not only sodium chloride as thought by many. Only 3 percent of the solution becomes tiny crystals that are barely visible in the laboratory glass. If sprayed over the skin, it is virtually impossible to appreciate them (imagine being able to see 3 percent of a micro drop from a spray). The main salts also include sodium carbonate/bicarbonate, magnesium chloride, magnesium sulfate, potassium chloride, calcium chloride, calcium hydroxide, calcium carbonate, potassium bromide and sulfurs (sodium sulfide) in combination with another element, especially a metal. Trace elements add significant properties to the ocean water since they remain in ionic form, which keeps them active for chemical reactions. They are called trace when compared with the major elements but their possible microbiological and metabolic activities do not require any specific volume. The bottom line is that the ions in ocean water are electrically charged and they continue to interact with each other, forming associations and separating at the same speed. These phenomena make the ocean a very unique element. The sea is a universe of chemical reactions impossible to decipher simply in a lifetime.

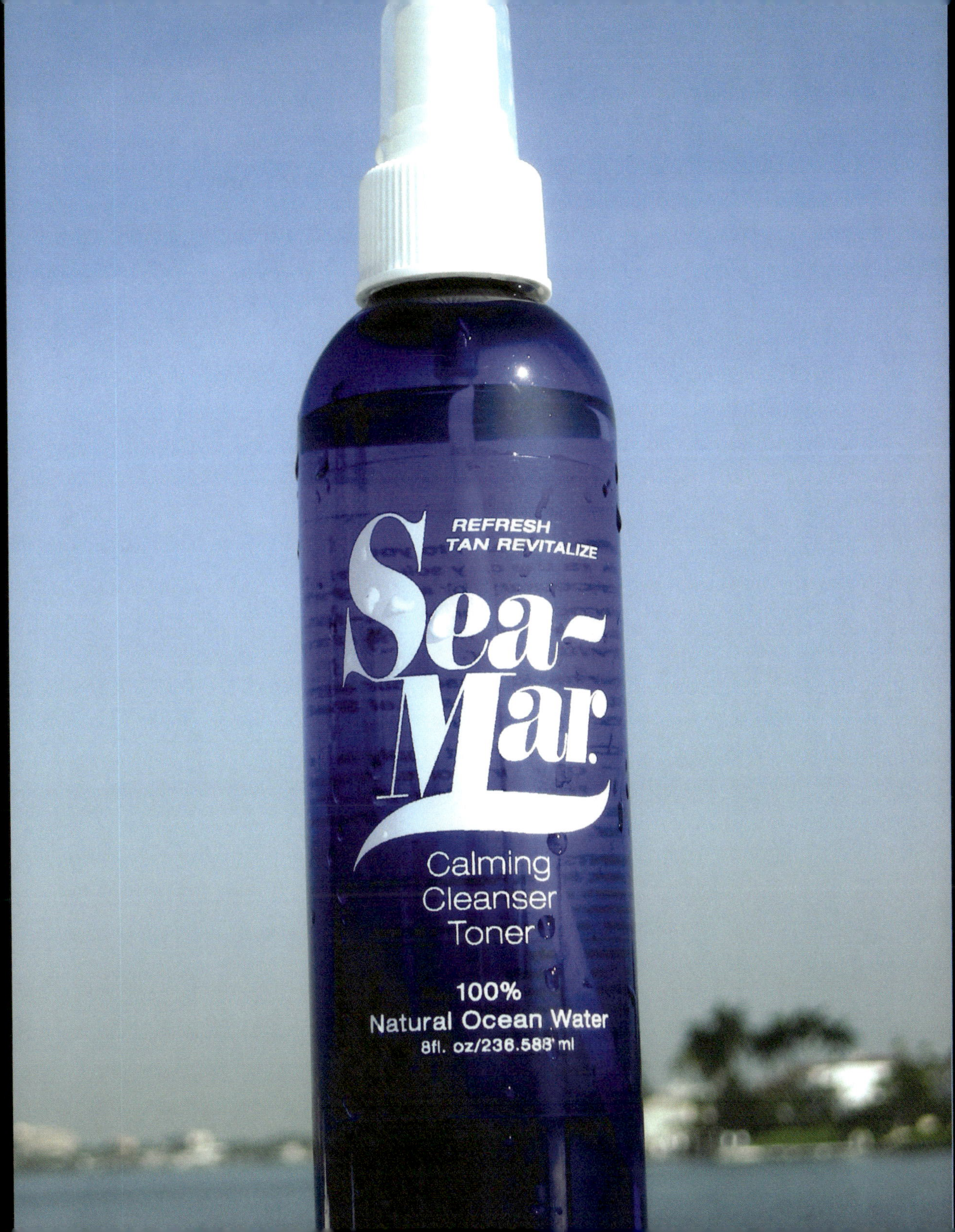
REFRESH
TAN REVITALIZE
Sea-Mar.
Calming
Cleanser
Toner
100%
Natural Ocean Water
8fl. oz/236.588 ml

After all, a Product named Sea~Mar®

Sea~Mar® does not cause any serious reaction in humans. It can be sprayed safely over the body causing just mild discomfort in the mucosa, particularly in the eyes, but significantly less than natural beach water. The solution is being tested multiple times before its final bottling for the consumer. The tests include highly sensitive and specific microbiological and chemical analyses. The immediate sensation reported by the consumers is of pleasure. **Sea~Mar®** is not recommended as a substitute for any medical treatment, and in case of a particular disease, you should always consult your doctor. The initial refreshing sensation is followed by one of soft tension or firmness due to the action of the ions dissolved. This sensation is also temporary and is finally followed by one of smooth and non-oily skin without taking away the natural radiance. **Sea~Mar®** has no chemicals added during the manufacturing process. It has no alcohol and no oil. It's odorless (fragrance free) and colorless, so there are no smells and no staining. The solution is noncomedogenic and it is compatible with any skin type.

The solution is obtained after raw ocean water is processed to remove all the plankton, sand, and all that which is not pure seawater on its natural ionic state. The process is completed by clean packaging that maintains the strict patented parameters. The quality control exceeds the requirements for the industry. Frequent testing is carried out and supervised by healthcare professionals.

Under magnification, the skin shows an immediate response to sprayed purified ocean water. A reduction in natural skin lines and skin folds has been photographed, but it is too early to classify the solution as an anti-wrinkle compound. These are the results of the opening of the water channels (aquaporins) and the ion channels of the cells in the epidermal layer, which is the most superficial aspect of the skin. In 2003, the Medicine Nobel Prize was awarded to Peter Agre and Roderick

Mckinnon for their works describing the function and structure of what is called the *aquaporins* (the water pores of the cells). Water channels in the human cells are also present in the skin cells. These water channels are activated by the ions present in solutions like purified ocean water that allow the hydration and possibly the revitalization of the skin cells. I have studied the effects of ions like the Sodium, Potassium, Chloride, and the Calcium ion. All of them individually open the ion channels, which allow the water penetration into the cells*. This novel concept moves today's cosmetic industry. *

(If you are a professional and would like to obtain more detailed information, do an online search in one of the popular Internet search engines for '*Seawater Aquaporins Regulation and Ion Channel Activity of a Solution Comprising Seawater;*' a scientific article should pop up.) Although there are no clinical trials on this specific product for psoriasis, acne or Atopic dermatitis, it wouldn't be surprising to find a similar result in the improvement already published and commented above.

The use of a name to identify a system is an old practice among scientists, doctors, and artists; however, the idea of mentioning my name to describe the method of application still sounds pompous to me. Anyway, it has to be called with a name—**The Soto System.**

The system involves purified ocean water, a fine mist spray, and a cosmetic action over the skin using specific directions to obtain each effect. The system to use **Sea~Mar**® as a cosmetic calculates the use of the fine mist spray applied on a specific range of seawater concentrations. The spray is located at different distances from the epidermis and it is pumped at different rates depending on the effects desired. An ancient method of applying different temperatures to the water before it is applied to the skin has been incorporated as well. This will be explained in more detail on the facial applications of seawater.

Mask and Primer

The benefit of a mask is the prolonged use of the sea minerals before and after the cosmetic. **Sea~Mar**® is used as a *primer* before applying cosmetics. The effect is a better adhesion of the cosmetics to the skin; possibly related to the opening of the water channels of the skin cells. Another evidence of the purified seawater refreshing effects is the better tolerance of the cosmetics on very sensitive facial skin. To use Sea~Mar as a *primer*, the purified ocean water should be lightly sprayed from five to ten inches from the face using the fine mist sprayer. **Sea~Mar** is also used as a revitalizer of the skin following other cosmetic uses. For example, to provide a maximum level of sea salt action, like using the **Sea~Mar**® fine mist spray, it's located closer to the skin, in a range of two inches, and it's pumped at least two times per area treated. This method causes a rapid skin hydration (moisturizing effect) and a high level of sea ions delivered per square inch. The solution is then left to dry over the skin to allow the absorption of the elements and the soft calming effect.

Toner

Dr. Soto's System also allows **Sea~Mar**® to be used as a skin toner. It's recommended to position the fine mist spray bottle at approximately five to ten inches from the skin. The pump is then activated twice over each area treated, and it produces a fresh mist of the ionic solution. This causes a different effect on the skin surface tension and sensations. The level of sea salt concentration is lower and the refreshing action is enhanced by the cooling effect of evaporation and the pharmacologically active salts.

The following pictures show a closer look of the skin's activity of **Sea-Mar**®. Before the action of the purified ocean water, the skin is dry and cracking, allowing the penetration of bacteria and irritants to the deeper structures. Once the solution is applied, the skin turned brighter, hydrated, and tended to close or made cracking disappear.

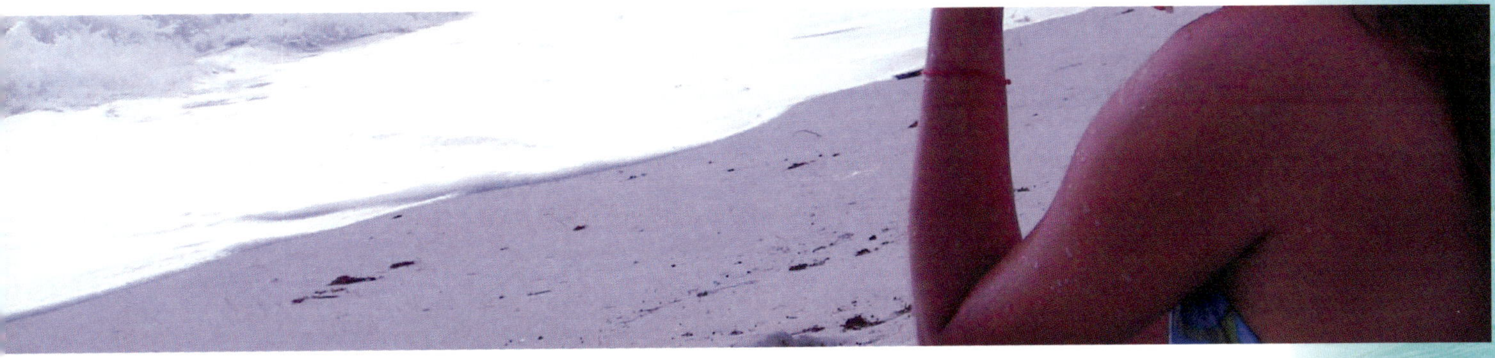

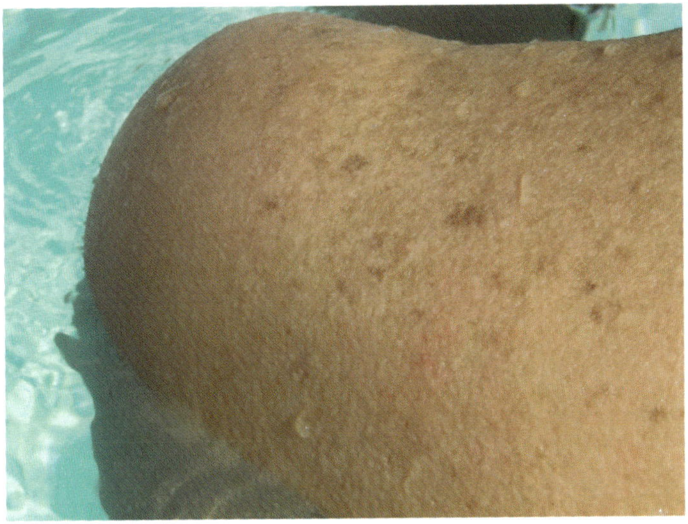

Sea Mask and Exfoliating Effects

To use **Sea~Mar**® as a sea mask, the spray is positioned at two inches from the skin and pressed three times per area of treatment to reach an appropriate level of minerals and trace elements at skin level. The liquid solution is left to dry on the skin and the smoothing effect follows. Using this modality, an exfoliating activity is expected by means of the sea salt action over the skin cells and the physical effect of the pressure gradient created by the pulses of gas and liquid generated by the pump over the stratus corneum of the skin.

Tanner

Nobody knows with certainty if going to the beach might give you a different pigmentation in the skin that, let's say is like going for a walk on a sunny day in Central Park, in New York City or to a sugar cane field in the island of Cuba. The general belief, however, is that the tan from the beach is different and much more special than simple exposure to the sun anywhere else.

There are scientific reasons to believe that seawater may stimulate a different level of tanning. The minerals present in the ocean water are able to penetrate and stick to the human cells. They probably have an action (particularly magnesium and calcium) stimulating the nucleus of the skin cells that causes the release of proteins by the melanocites. Melanocite are those cells responsible for the color of our skin and melanin needs specific stimulation through proteins that act as messengers for their release. The process takes days and the skin color will continue to accent in the days after the beach visit. This is scientific theory. It could be definitely tested any of these days considering the technology available to quantify skin coloration. One sure thing is that the minerals in the ocean water really penetrate the superficial skin structures and may be deeper.

Sea~Mar® is used as a tanner. The fine mist spray is applied as much as desired by the users; however, it is recommended always to apply a sunblocker or sunscreen before to prevent skin cancer and to avoid serious sunburns due to excessive irradiation with ultraviolet light. The solution can be safely applied as much as needed to evoke a cooling sensation while being on the pool, the beach, or the tanning salon. In this case, the tan at New York Central Park might be just as beautiful as the one in Cape Cana in the Dominican Republic or in Ibiza, Spain.

This modality allows the immediate moisturizing effect of the ocean water. A pleasant refreshing sensation and a toning action is the result of this form of application. The advantage of the different forms of this new system is that they facilitate frequent repetitions over time that allow the skin to remain smooth, moisturized, and facilitating the absorption of key minerals and trace elements through the epidermis in an ionic way.

Sea~Mar® does not cause any skin tanning if the person is not exposed enough to the sun or ultraviolet radiation. In this way, the incidental tanning effect is very minimal and ultimately depends on the amount of the radiation exposure.

Ocean water	Chloride: Cl	Potassium: K	Sodium: Na	Magnesium Mg	Calcium Ca	Sulfate S
Human body	**The most common electrolyte in the body**	**The most important electrolyte inside the human cells**	**The most important ion outside the human cells. Key element for human cell hydration**	**Also considered a chemical messenger and the key ion for skin disease treatments**	**It's necessary for the cells' activities and it is also a chemical messenger**	**It's a key ingredient for many dermatological compounds due to its activity in the skin. It's part of the ions necessary for the cell's metabolism**

II) Spa and *Thalassotherapy* Applications

Sanus Per Aquam (SPA) or Sanitas Per Aquas. That is the origin of the word *spa* in the Roman times. According to Rohan Mistry, PhD, the soldiers exhausted by the wars were taken to rejuvenation and relaxing baths in hot spring waters. Caracalla Baths are another example of the luxurious baths built by the Romans and able to host hundreds of people at a time. The combination of the benefits of the bath and the social gathering made these places a favorite of this ancient culture. The *spa* was the other alternative in recreation compared to the Roman Circus Massimo and the Coliseum, but they also shared common grounds. Next to the ruins of the Roman Coliseum can be seen what the gladiator's pool was then. This was a bath to be used by those winning the battles at the arena. The gladiators probably felt so well that they chose nothing better after the battles than the healing touch of the water.

The typical Roman spa had common features that have survived to our days and marked a style in the services. According to the research done by Liberati and Bourbon, the first room in the "baths" was the changing room followed by the hot bath room, then a moderately heated room, and finally the cold bath pool. The spa was always the center of peace and balance. The first world's spas were probably adorned with flowers, sweet perfumes, and nicely colored drapes. The ambience was appropriate for massages, saunas, and depilation. There was space for libraries, a gymnasium, lounges, and even areas for dining, like fast food places. It was definitely in the midst of an atmosphere necessary to create a perfect social gathering, to propose business, and to deliver encouraging messages. The water was in the center of the happening.

Unfortunately, the spa tradition and its benefits disappeared with time. At the end of the nineteenth century and the beginning of the twentieth, the spa tradition was reborn. The advances in clinical medicine, rehabilitation, surgery, orthopedic and the explosion of new technology made feasible this resurging. In the United States, spas have a routine presence in big hotels and cruise liners. It's possible now to enjoy the benefits of the bath and the relaxing atmosphere without regard to the weather. The spa might be in the hub or in the cruise; you just need to find it.

Sea~Mar® is used also as spa product. It has been proven that the solution applied in the form of aerosol on the face and other parts of the human body produce excellent results. When nebulized over the skin, the micro drops tend to aggregate, forming bigger drops and they are better absorbed through the skin's pores. The effect is an immediate hydration of the skin surface and softening of the stratus corneum, which is composed mostly of dead cells. The solution can be used first as a cleanser to prepare the skin for the treatment, or it can be applied as the only therapy using all the seawater properties. Below you can find a brief description of how we recommend that you apply the product in the salon. It's recommended to have at least two bottles—one is used at the spa treatment area; the other one is to be kept cold and stored inside a refrigerator while not in use.

Tanning by the Pool or in the Chamber:

Sea-Mar® can be used as a tanner; however, this is based on the general belief that ocean water helps to acquire a tan different than what can be obtained in a lake or when a person is exposed by the pool at home. As expressed before, the combination of minerals and trace elements might justify such a belief due to the possible stimulating activity of such elements on the cellular metabolism. The use of Sea-Mar in the tanning salon is gaining popularity and at least the refreshing and smoothing effects over the skin are undeniable.

Sea-Mar can be used before and during tanning sessions by spraying the compound over the areas. Press the pump from about five to ten inches from the skin.

Dr. Soto Sea Water Facial

First, the recipient of the treatment should be placed in a comfortable position with the head resting on a couch or a chair with head support. Cover the hair if you wish to avoid undesired effects of the solution on a recently done hairstyle. The eyes should be covered with small 2x2 gauzes. Start the procedure.

1) Humidify the skin using a fine mist aerosol machine with warm seawater at 38°C. Apply enough purified seawater to allow the formation of micro-drops on the face. This process takes an average of ten minutes. It's called *humectation* and it is intended for the initial softening of the skin and opening of the pores.

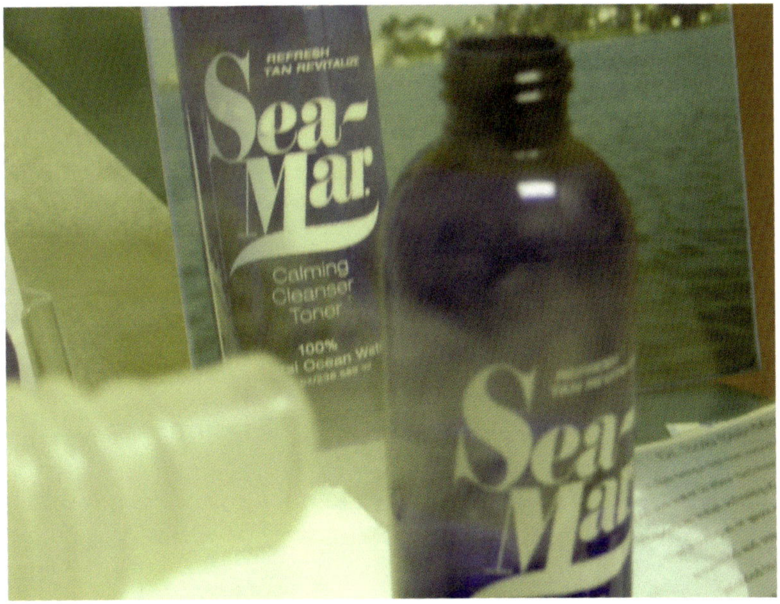

2) Use a soft pad or gauze embedded with **Sea~Mar** ® to gently remove the makeup, dust particles, excess oil, and superficial dead cells using circular movements. It's called the *exfoliation* phase. It's intended to reduce the number of dead cells and expose the younger layer of skin. Average time is three minutes.

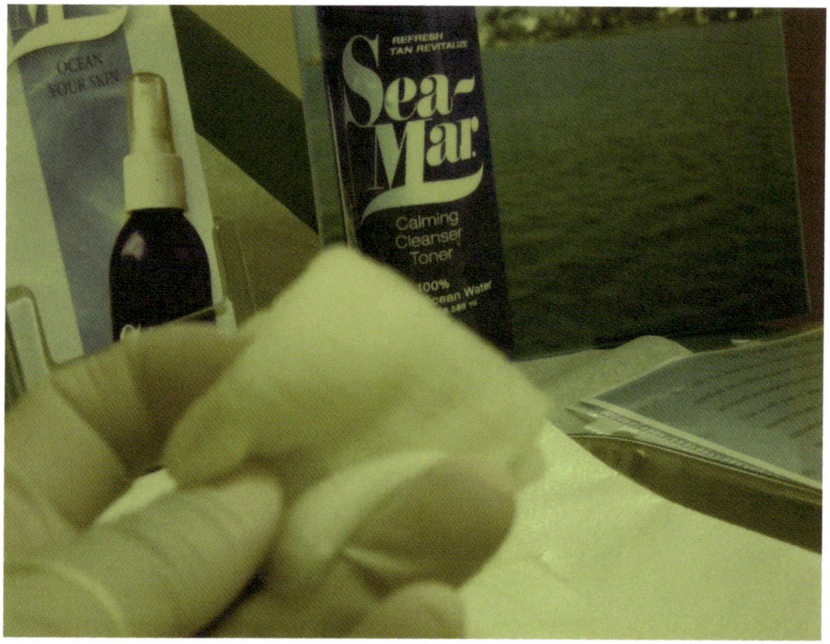

3) Apply a second dose of the misting solution to allow a deeper penetration of the key minerals and the trace elements on the skin. This process is called trans-mineralization. It's intended to facilitate the penetration of minerals necessary for a healthy skin. This phase lasts for about ten minutes.

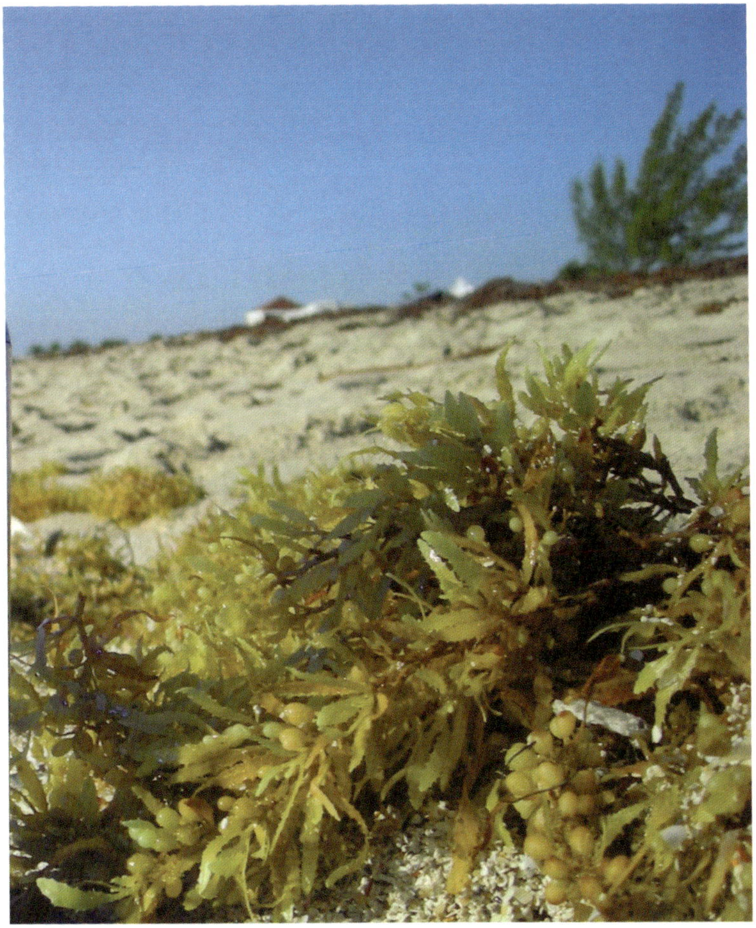

4) The skin is now ready for a massage using a roll-on or a vibrating device over the face. The facial can be done using mild pressure applied with the fingers pads. The rubbing should be applied in the traditional face massage technique using a circular movement and frequent additions of purified seawater. Always be gentle and make movements of the fingers from the back to the center of the face and ascending to

complete a full circle. The fingers or devices stimulate the blood circulation at skin level and increases the mineral penetration to deeper skin structures. This process lasts about ten minutes.

5) **If no other substances have been applied, then skip this step**. Apply **Sea~Mar** ® as a cleanser using a soft pad; once again to eliminate residuals of other substances used by the skin care specialist. This process lasts about two minutes.

6) Apply cold **Sea~Mar** ® in the form of spray from about ten inches from the skin using two puffs per area. The temperature of the purified ocean water should be between 4 and 9 Celsius degree. This process lasts approximately one minute or less.

7) Gently rinse the face with tap water to avoid sticky eyelashes; one minute or less. Total of the average time is thirty-eight minutes or more.

Thalassotherapy—The Old and the New Marine Therapy

The International Federation of Thalassotherapy, Sea and Health (*Federation Internationale de Thalasotherapie, Mer et Sante)* gives the following definition about marine therapy: ***"In a privileged place, Thalassotherapy is the simultaneous use, under normal medical supervision, with a preventive goal, of the benefit of the marine environment that involves the marine climate, the seawater, the marine mud and other sea substances"*** (updated on March, 2008 *www.thalassofederation.com*).

Phytotherapy—Therapy with Algae

Some advantages of the plants grown in the ocean are that they don't require fertilizers to stimulate their growth. There is absolutely no need to use pesticides, and the contents of calcium, iron and trace elements is high. Algae are used in the spa in a variety of forms depending on their type. It's said they help to preserve skin hydration and facilitate the penetration of trace elements through the skin. Algae's active principles (chemical components with a known effect) are considered as excellent skin toners. According to Riad Dikes and Vincent Gallon, new research has demonstrated excellent active properties of seaweeds and algae. It's said, for example, that algae of the *Laminaria* genus have sebum-regulating properties. The same applies to *Chondrus crispus*, also known as Irish or carrageen moss, which is a source of a polysaccharide. *Rhodymenia palmate* is red seaweed that grows on rocks in the oceans and contains multiple vitamins. *Ulva lactuca* (sea lettuce) has cosmetic properties. It may also stimulate the production of collagen and elastin.

Allergies or contact dermatitis, however, have been reported. The same adverse effect could be expected from the use of creams with algae ingredients due to algae and the preservatives used in the industry.

Hydro-massage

Hydro-massage is probably the broadest name for a number of different treatments using seawater as the common element. Definitely, *thalassotherapy* would be even more specific, but it's still too broad to know they're referring to. That's why I like the use of very direct names for therapy modalities that allow a closer range of definitions.

Seawater Massage

Seawater can be used for massage therapy. The hydrostatic pressure could help to stimulate the blood and lymphatic circulation in the human body. Hydrostatic pressure is the natural pressure caused by the liquid over a surface, in this case the body. It's believed that this physical phenomena ultimately causes stimulation of the digestive process favoring the natural intestinal movement and a diuretic effect that helps the kidneys to function. The natural ocean water massage is relaxing. The sound of the waves is rhythmic, slow, and frequently at a low volume. All these conditions favor a natural hypnotic effect that helps you to relax.

Flotation and Flotarium

A *flotarium* is an area dedicated to the principle of flotation with therapeutic intentions. In other words, floating on the water might have benefits to human health. The human body weighs significantly less in ocean water. Sometimes the weight is up to a tenth of its real value under normal gravity conditions. This special condition allows the patients of the practice to use the normal sea conditions by the beach as the ideal environment to regain strength of debilitated muscles, painful joints or injured areas. Although this needs to be done under specific medical guidance, the process of recovery is facilitated by the near weightlessness conditions found in the ocean, the soft bottom of the sandy beaches, the continuous massage of the waves, the hypnotic sound, and the nicest views on earth. Of course, this process can be replicated in specialized facilities far from the beaches, and even modern equipment can be included to combine more than one modality of treatment.

Jet Stream and Showers

Frequently interpreted and accepted as *hydro-massage,* t he uses of jet power in spas is disseminated worldwide. The water jets and showers are located in bathroom areas or open pools. Probably it all started during the medieval times near the town fountain, the public Roman bath, or the aqueducts. The result is that gravity and water combined form a stream. The impact of the stream in the body has been described as beneficial in many ways. Blood circulation is directly affected by the effects of the stream over the blood vessels as well as over the big group of muscles, which contains significant amounts of blood.

A separate effect is the action over the muscles' fibers and the nerve endings that produce a direct relaxing effect and pain relief in conditions such as sport injuries, muscle tension, arthritis, and degenerative joint disease. The jet stream produces different effects and sensations depending on the length of the exposure to the treatment, the stream speed, and the stream volume. The shape of the stream may have an impact in how the treatment is perceived; however, the speed and the volume of water are more determinant factors in the results.

Watsu

Watsu is a modality of stream used under water combined with the traditional *Shiatsu* as a modality of deep massage to stimulate nerves and deeper structures. *Watsu* was invented by an American, H. Dull as a form of relaxation.

Hydrothermal Pools

Seawater is frequently heated to a temperature acceptable to the human body. Heated ocean water stimulates an increase in the lymphocytes type eight. These particular cells are responsible for decreasing the type of immune reactions that cause inflammation, so the effect of heated seawater would be anti-inflammatory. It has been proven in Japan that deep seawater has a beneficial effect on patients affected by Atopic Dermatitis (AD).

Hydrothermal pools are also effective to promote muscle and mental relaxation. The increase in the water temperature improves the blood circulation by a phenomenon called *vasodilatation* where the blood vessels open up and the red blood cells can reach areas normally poorly irrigated. The cascade of events allows better oxygenation of muscles, cartilages, and bones. The toxic substances normally accumulated in these areas can then be removed by the improved blood stream and exchange of substances. All of the above events contribute to pain reduction or elimination, improve muscle activity, and increase the range of motion for the joints if combined with exercise.

Hydrokynesotherapy

Like a gym in the water, *hydrokynesotherapy* is a long, long word invented to say just that—exercises in the water. I recommend to some of my patients that they submerge themselves with the shoulders slightly under the water, so the four extremities are relaxed. Using this method, the muscles are exposed to a higher resistance. The impact is almost zero. In this form of therapy, the muscle strength is developed without traumatic effect over the bones or cartilages. It's an ideal training modality for older people, and of course, for Olympic swimmers. It's estimated that the caloric consumption is higher (double) for the same type of exercises inside the water. In other words, you can obtain the same or better results doing the exercises just half of the time inside a pool or in the water by the beach.

A current popular trend is pool aerobics and they are practiced in many hotels in the Dominican Republic, Club Med, and other resorts for which medical supervision might not be requested.

Jacuzzi

In 1968, Roy Jacuzzi invented the *Jacuzzi®*, the first whirlpool bath, totally self-contained. The Jacuzzi family started the whirlpool bath using a barrel, and the Jacuzzi brings pleasure and healing to many families. It's essentially just like that original idea—a bathtub with "water that moves you." The water might be heated or at a regular temperature. It can be combined with essential oils, perfumes, soaps and even music and colorful lights. The effects over the physical well-being are incredibly rewarding. A hydromassage of this type, especially if it is done with warm seawater, has a direct effect over the circulation. In addition, it decreases muscle pain and helps people suffering from tendonitis, arthritis, lower back pain and foot pain.

A perfect length of time to experience a Jacuzzi type of bath is twenty minutes. Of course, it can be longer or you may choose to alternate periods of streaming jets and quiet time to enjoy the bubble stimulation of the skin receptors, which I found to be very relaxing. Longer periods may predispose you to dehydration or a decrease in blood pressure that might be dangerous.

The use of seawater or chemical elements such as soap and aromatic oils, indicates the need for a rinsing shower after the event. If this is the case, make sure that the temperature of the shower water is the same that was used in the bathtub, so the relaxing effect lasts longer.

Marine Sauna

Vapors of volcanic origin can be found in the natural vents at great depths in the ocean. These vapors can be lethal to humans if we were exposed to them. However, modern therapy has come up with the revolutionary method of marine vapors using heated seawater.

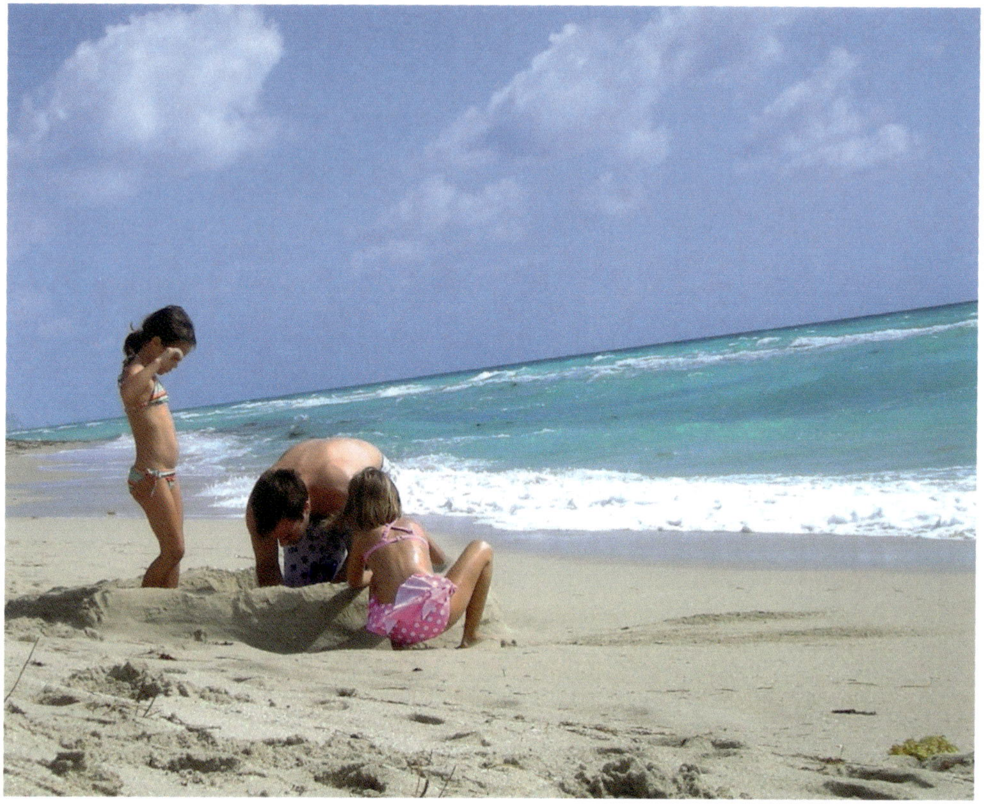

Sand therapy

(*Arenoterapia*) is the use of sand to obtain health benefits or for cosmetic purposes. The uses of sand can be extraordinary due to the plasticity of this compound. Sand is composed mostly of silicon. Its texture and variety allows multiple uses. Sand is a product of erosion. Its color might go from almost white, through different yellow tones, and then through black. There are at least two places in the world with black sands—the first, Bibijagua Beach (pronounced like *bebehawoa)* in the Isla de la Juventud (Youth Island) in Cuba, south of the Habana province. The second is in Costa Rica. Sand is also used as a psychological instrument to produce relaxation through activities due to its physical properties. Sand is valuable for children and adults who simply want to play with it. Sand figures modeling (castle, channel, bodies, faces, objects, etc.) might be just a change to a simpler and distracting activity. The psychological benefits include relaxation and extinguishing undesired behavioral patterns. Sand is also applied warm over the body to produce a tactile saturation of the senses and to cause a light exfoliating effect. This property allows the removal of dead cells from the skin surface and cleans the more superficial layer.

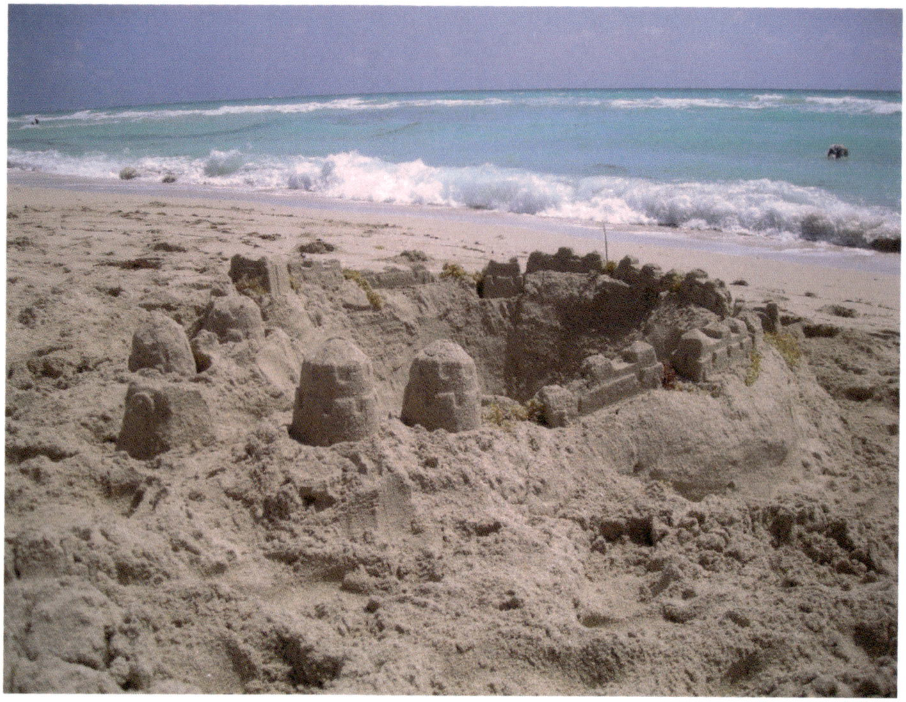

Modeling and playing with sand claim our concentration and help us to break away from odd thoughts and stressful ideas. Children with psychological problems may manifest certain behavioral changes when exposed to sand and may express symptoms like tics or disruptive behavior after or during the exposure to this natural element. The consult with a psychologist is definitely one to consider. Sand therapy as a psychological tool is valuable when guided by an experienced psychologist. As a cosmetic or Thalassotherapy alternative, it might be applied as a scrub, moist or dry, warm or at room temperature, all over the body or in certain areas only. There is no doubt of the clear benefits in the skin and the mind.

Liquid sound is another trend and there is a good reason for it.

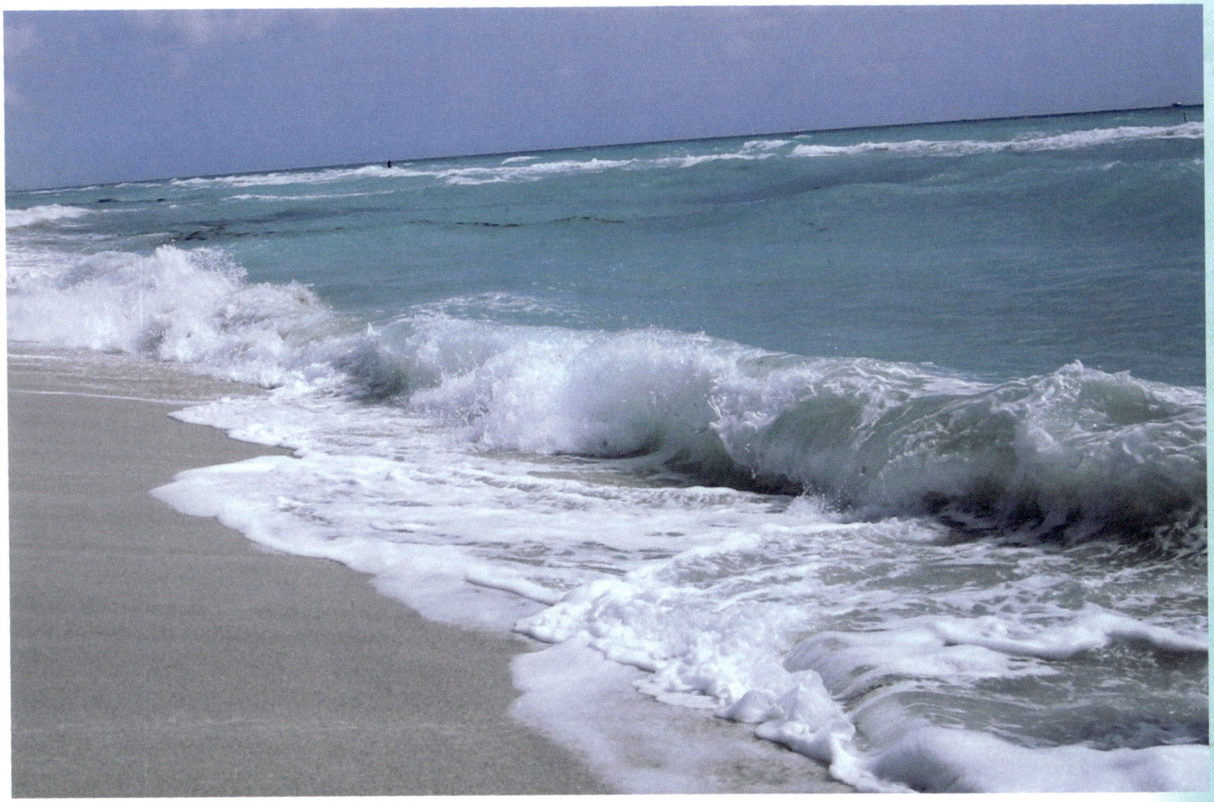

Water sounds have very special effects in the human mind. I have seen therapists using a common rainy day as a perfect background for a relaxing therapy session. Try this if you are so lucky and you're caught at home on a rainy day. Close your eyes and focus on the sound of the water drops and streams falling beyond the walls of your room. Listen to every drop if you can. Imagine the bubbles, the colors, the temperature, and the sensation of the warm water falling through your skin. You might find this relaxing and invigorating. You may even fall sleep. It's not coincidental that many hotels, restaurants, palaces, and convention centers have water fountains as an ornament in certain places; it's the water.

Dead Sea and Marine Mud

The Dead Sea is located at 31°20′N 35°30′E, between Israel and Jordan. An entire city could be built on its bottom. It's about 800 Km² (some 300 square miles). It was part of the sea in the past, but eventually became trapped and isolated from the rest of the ocean. The Dead Sea is the lowest surface point on earth. That means that without descending beyond the surface of the soil, this would be the lowest point on the planet, just as the tip of Mount Everest would be the highest point. Lake Asal, in Somalia has similar characteristics, but Lake Asal is even saltier than the Dead Sea. Great Salt Lake, in Utah, United States, also has a very high salinity.

The Dead Sea is actually a lake. It's covered by water which is extremely salty, thicker in texture, and is extraordinarily beneficial for the human skin when it's used properly. Several scientific researchers have concluded that the effects of the sea salts are evident during diseases like Psoriasis and Atopic Dermatitis. The heavy salt content makes anybody easily float on its waters. There is also mud that might have additional health effects. The mud is used today in the cosmetic industry and is easily found on the Internet at various web sites.

The chemical composition of the Dead Sea water has the same six key elements of the ocean, but with much higher concentrations; sometime forming crystals of chemical compounds. This particular aspect makes the Dead Sea raw materials more favorable for lotions and creams. Dead Sea mud contains minerals and can be applied warm or at room temperature. The natural raw material is combined these days with other elements by specialists in the industry which allows combined effects like hydration and revitalization of the skin and even wrinkle reduction as recently claimed. The benefits of the bath in the Dead Sea have been related to the level of ultraviolet radiation measured at the Dead Sea. The sun's radiation is lower than in other areas of the planet, so the skin effects are probably better.

Dr. I. Machtey studied the influences of Dead Sea Bath Salts on rheumatic patients suffering from osteoarthritis or a localized type of tendonitis. One-hundred and three patients were treated for one or two weeks with daily use of the Dead Sea Bath Salts in a sanatorium located in the Dead Sea about 400 m above sea level. The improvement was impressive. The greater the limitations of the patients, the better they progressed. The study was published as *"Dead Sea Balneotherapy in Osteoarthritis," Dr. Machtey (Hasharon Hospital, Petach-Tikya, Isreal).* Published in Proceedings of International Seminar on Treatment of Rheumatic Diseases," John Wright, PSG, Inc. (1982).

Similar studies have been done in Europe. Dr. J. Arndt from Germany made a study of the effect of Dead Sea Bath Salts on patients suffering from psoriasis. Fifty patients, aged between fourteen and seventy-seven years were treated with the salts in a controlled way. Treatment consisted of partial or total baths. For a total bath, two Kgs of the salts were dissolved in a bath at a temperature of 27 C. The partial baths were made with a concentration of about 10 percent. The baths lasted for twenty minutes and afterwards the skin was thoroughly rinsed with running water. The effect was enhanced when the patient remained in a warm packed condition for one hour after the bath. The study was published as *"Salt from the Promised Land Helps Psoriasis Patients," Dr. J. Arndt, Published in Arztliche Praxis, vol. 34, No. 48, 1920,(15.6.1982).*

Similar studies have been done in other parts of the world. All of them bring to light the same scientific conclusion—the sea salts are healing if they are applied properly and supervised by a specialist.

It's imperative that the persons interested in this type of therapy consult with their family doctor before engaging in any of these treatments, particularly if they suffer from cardiovascular conditions like coronary artery disease, hypertension, or cerebrovascular disease.

The possibility of its application as a registered product through regulatory agencies like the Food and Drug Administration in the United States is being considered. The cosmetic aspect, however, is definitely one already tried by many generations. The scientific community and ultimately the general public have the final word.

III) Psychological Effects of the Sea Elements

We have talked before about the successful application of sand therapy by psychologists, but let's talk now about the other elements. The neuro-psychological effects of ocean water in humans have been analyzed by different authors. The common ground is that there is a positive impact in the human behavior or at least in the human response to the exposure to marine environments under appropriate circumstances. Let's start by saying that the ocean sounds, for example, are considered what is called a "primordial sound;" those sounds produced by humans or nature that can be formatted in certain ways to produce a deep effect in the human mind and behavior. It has been proven that these kinds of sounds have evident results when they are produced, for example, in a repetitive way and at low intensity—just like the waves breaking softly on a sandy beach, in a calm day. The sound is perceived by the human brain as a calming sound...but why? (Always *why?*)

The human brain produces electrical waves as part of its normal functioning. This has been extensively studied by scientists all over the world for many years. An *electroencephalogram (EEG)* is a test normally done in a hospital or clinic to evaluate these brain electrical waves. Well, some of these waves are related to intense brain activity and others have more *calming* functions. The ***Beta*** waves relate to thinking, mind and body activity. They have a frequency measured in the EEG at 14 to 30 Hz. Not a coincidence, the ocean waves under calm conditions produce sounds between 0.05 to 16 Hz. This means that we probably vibrate in the same frequency as the ocean. If we're exposed long enough, we might feel calmer and much more relaxed. Rhythmic and repetitive sounds from the ocean water at low intensity might have an impact in the human's natural trend to think, meditate and possibly to cause a sense of calm. The benefit might start almost immediately after the exposure to the source of the sound, in this case, the ocean itself. The sound, however, might be recorded and reproduced later in a room, even during several sessions. These sounds might help to induce sleep. If all these things happen through sounds, then what would be the effect of submerging a human body in this electro-magnetic field that is the seawater?

I am also fascinated with the extraordinary forms of energy transmission in the universe—everything is through *waves*—sound waves, brain waves, light waves, pressure waves, and of course, sea waves.

Japanese scientists Choi Jong-in, Hota Kenji and Yamazaki Ken, have studied the influences of the reproduction of wave sounds in the functioning and mind activity of the human body. They have recently published something astonishing. After their scientific analysis, they have concluded that the ultrasonic sounds (those sounds not even heard by humans) that form part of the coastal waves have an effect on human brain waves. Some testimonies are clear in the sense of inspiration produced by staying or walking near the ocean. Some reported that it helps to arrive at problem resolution and that it helps to reprocess information stored in the subconscious. However, don't accept everything I have said in this chapter. Try it yourself.

There are abundant forms of recorded ocean sounds in the market these days. You can find recordings combining natural ocean sounds with music or even the ocean sounds alone. Some materials involve seagull sounds, harps, organ music and soft bells, piano and other elements that produce relaxing sensations.

A twenty-minute walk by the beach or near the shores might be as good as a talk with a good friend. Of course, I believe that human voice is another "primordial sound" and for many reasons irreplaceable. Interest studies done with human speech alone showed that when recordings of people speaking were speeded up, they sounded like birds chirping. However, when they were slowed down, they sounded like dolphins or like the flow of the ocean (www.bodymind.com). Dr. Jeffrey Thompson has described NASA recordings of outer space reflected sounds, picked within the range of human hearing, while the *Voyager* was passing by the outer planets of the solar system—Jupiter, Saturn, Uranus and Neptune. "*They sound remarkably like ocean sounds, dolphins, and birds.*"

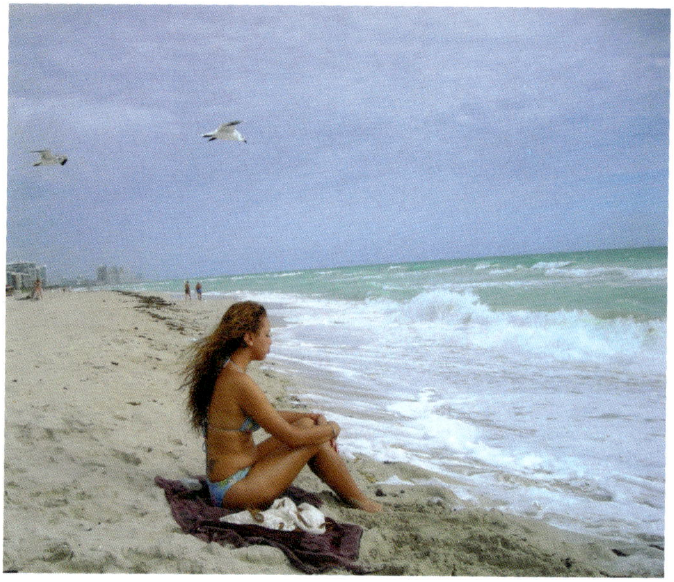

Walking along the beach is a perfect combination of healthy elements—the physical exercise is matched by a high level of oxygenation and the abundant negative ions present within a mile from the coastal line. The presence of sunlight is excellent for the human mind against depression. Sunlight is also necessary for vitamin D production to promote stronger bones. The natural beauty of the sight is added to the list of benefits, and then, the sounds and the body feelings of the wind and the ocean water itself. Take off your shoes if you can and experience a natural foot massage together with the exfoliation of all the undesired calluses. Splash water if is not too cold. Submerge yourself if is warm enough to do so. Just be careful and don't overdo it. Safety and balance are the key words. Pleasure and good health must be the goals all the time.

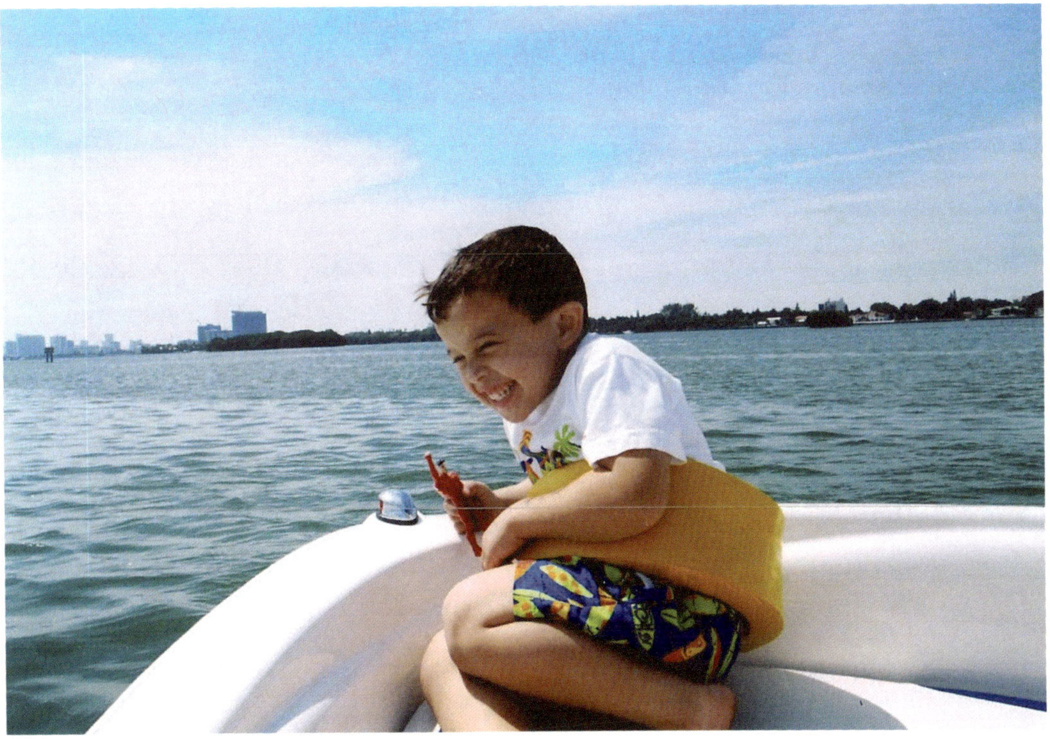

IV) Respiratory Diseases

The findings of the cosmetic effects followed an earlier discovery. A solution made from ocean water can be used for the treatment of respiratory diseases. The studies started in the city of Surfside, Florida in the year 2003 after a trip to the beach located in the 90th Street to collect the first gallon of seawater to be used for the experiment. I went with my older son who was seven years old at the time, for the tradition of good luck that connects the kids and the ocean.

Our home was within walking distance of the beach and when I returned, the experiment started. I filtered the water several times in the eyes of my incredulous wife until a grade of purity was achieved. Part of the resulting solution was sent to the laboratory for chemical and microbiological analysis; the rest went to an aerosol machine to experiment its nebulization. The event was documented in the notebook and the feasibility of the process enlightened that night and many others ahead. The process would open doors for people all over the world who suffered from asthma, bronchitis, emphysema, Atelectasis, common colds, or even other less common problems but as severe as cystic fibrosis.

I rushed to describe the method. I conducted two independent patent searches—one by myself, and the other one by the Calder Library at the University of Miami/Jackson Memorial Hospital. I contacted an attorney's firm and worked many nights to bring to light the solution and its proportions. The process was long and costly. More than four years of discussions, paperwork and a tedious wait for the patent examination. I applied for a second patent as an extension of the initial findings. The patent was rigidly examined. It was challenged more than once. Some of the claims were removed. I prepared corrections and clarified my point of view about the discovery and the usefulness. I waited until May 17, 2006. One afternoon, while on the phone with my father who was living in Havana, Cuba, I received a call from the attorneys at Sanchelima and Associates firm. "The patent was approved by the United States Patent and Trademark Office in Washington D.C." It was my wife's birthday.

I ran to the backyard and jumped on "La Niña," my little boat. I praised God for the achievement. Then I rinsed my face and my head with ocean water from the bow, like the Neptunian tradition for the young sailors.

United States Patent and Trademark Office Patent 7097852

The patent was developed based on the experiences of the author as early as 2003. The patent is not all inclusive, but it gives a perfect idea of the concept. In spite of the numerous jokes I have heard, I have to clarify that I am not attempting to patent the sea, but the clear concept of purification and medical use for respiratory diseases in aerosol. With this process the resulting highly purified ocean water can be packed and made available for its use under any weather or distance from the shores. This is not the first time that seawater has been taken as the original matter to develop a solution, but the end solution itself is different. The method of application and purposes are radically novel.

The cosmetic uses of the solution although envisioned were not patented by then, but trademarked, which made more economical sense by the time this was developed. Most of the description of the patent is made in a communicative way for someone who is not versed in the topic.

Solution comprising seawater as expectorant and virucidal for the treatment of respiratory diseases and method to use and develop.

Patent Number 7097852. Primary Class 424/439

International Class A61K9/00; A61K9/08; A61K9/12

Patent Filing date 8/18/2003: Publication 8/ 29/ 2006

Inventor: Jose Antonio Soto, M.D.

Abstract of Dr. Soto's Patent

A solution comprised of filtered natural seawater comprising pharmaceutically active salts and trace elements having a direct effect in the respiratory tissues and secretions as expectorant, mucolytic, decongestant and virucidal. Aerosolized treatment of the solution for a patient in need thereof dehydrates tissue, destroys mucous plugs, and mobilizes phlegm in the respiratory tract. A method of preparing the solution comprises extracting seawater from a depth beyond where microscopic organisms known as plankton lives, in an ocean; filtering said seawater to obtain desired concentration of elements; testing said seawater for microbiological and chemical analysis; and preparing the solution for packaging, having a predetermined approximated seawater element content as expectorant, mucolytic, decongestant, and virucidal.

What is claimed is:

1. A therapeutic solution comprised of filtered seawater in the form of an aerosolized solution in the respiratory tract of mammals; said therapeutic solution having a direct effect in respiratory tissues and secretions as expectorant, mucolytic and decongestant wherein said filtered seawater comprises approximately from 277.00 to 555.00 millimoles per liter of sodium, 417.00 to 894.00 millimoles per liter of chloride, 9.80 to 11.70 millimoles per liter of potassium, 20.90 to 26.13 millimoles per liter of sulfate, 45.60 to 60.49 millimoles per liter of magnesium, and 8.11 to 10.87 millimoles per liter of calcium, wherein osmolality is from 920 to 1,130 mOsml/Kg and pH is between 5.7 and 6.8.
2. The therapeutic solution set forth in claim 1, further characterized in that said therapeutic solution is administered by aerosol to said respiratory tract of said mammals such that said therapeutic solution contacts areas where said mucosa secretions accumulate including nose, pharynx, larynx, trachea, bronchi, bronchioles and alveoli.

V) The therapeutic solution set forth in claim 2, further characterized in that said therapeutic solution is administered by nebulization with a dose of approximately between one to ten ml via nasal or oral cavity to reach intratracheobronchial tissues and secretions with a varying frequency of administration according to said mammals age group and clinical diagnosis, said nebulization every two to twelve hours and extending three to fifteen minutes, said therapeutic solution may be administered in a dry form through inhalations of one to three per time.

1. The therapeutic solution set forth in claim 2, further characterized in that said therapeutic solution is administered with tents or a vaporization system in a continuous form for up to twenty-four hours.
2. A method for treating respiratory tissues and secretions as expectorant, mucolytic and decongestant in a mammal in need thereof, comprising administering to said mammal an effective amount of a therapeutic solution as set forth in claim 1, said therapeutic solution comprised of filtered seawater and administered in the form of an aerosolized solution via nasal or oral cavity by nebulization with a dose of approximately between one to ten ml. with varying frequency of administration according to said mammal's age group and clinical diagnosis, said nebulization administered every two to twelve hours, extending three to fifteen minutes to reach intratracheobronchial tissues and secretions and said solution increases the solubility and volume of the phlegm in a respiratory tract reducing the adhesiveness and making them easier to expel by means of coughing or suctioning, providing a symptomatic relief of cough and congestion associated with bronchial asthma, acute and chronic bronchitis and common colds, and wherein said solution increases output of said secretions from said respiratory tract by stimulating ciliary movement which facilitates the removal of mucus and said solution stimulates water transport into an airway lumen to decrease the inflammatory changes in a respiratory tree

associated with bronchial asthma, chronic bronchitis and common colds.

3. The solution set forth in claim 2 wherein said solution is used as a vehicle for delivering drugs into the respiratory tract of a mammal.

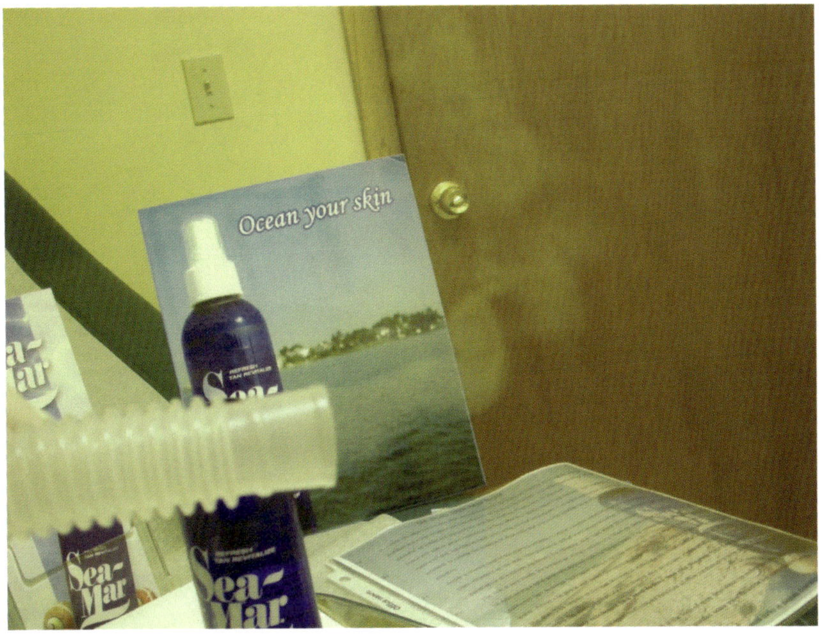

The instant invention is also a method of preparing a therapeutic solution, comprising:

A) extracting seawater from a depth beyond where microscopic organisms known as plankton lives, in an ocean;

B) filtering said seawater to obtain desired concentration of elements; said elements primarily comprising sodium, magnesium, calcium, potassium, chloride, and sulfate;

C) testing said seawater for microbiological and chemical analysis; and

D) preparing a solution for packaging, having a predetermined approximated seawater element content as expectorant, mucolytic, decongestant, and virucidal.

It's therefore one of the main objects of the present invention to provide a solution made of filtered natural seawater comprising pharmaceutically active salts and trace elements that have a direct effect in respiratory tissues and secretions when administered.

It's another object of this invention to provide a solution made of filtered natural seawater comprising pharmaceutically active salts and trace elements that are an expectorant, mucolytic, decongestant and have a virucidal effect when administered.

It's another object of the present invention to provide a solution made of filtered natural seawater comprising pharmaceutically active salts and trace elements, for solution aerosol administration in the form of vials.

It's yet another object of the present invention to provide a solution having a low acid pH that allows viral penetration through cellular walls, into the cytoplasm of a cell.

It's still another object of this invention to provide such a solution that is inexpensive to manufacture and administer while retaining its effectiveness.

Further objects of the invention will be brought out in the following part of the specification, wherein detailed description is for the purpose of fully disclosing the invention without placing limitations thereon.

The type of the trace elements will vary with the seawater origin, so may its concentration. The solvent for the solution is the seawater. The compounds of the invention, as well as the pharmaceutically acceptable salts thereof, due to the pharmacological properties and very low toxicity can be used as active ingredients for the preparation of *medicaments* for the respiratory diseases.

After testing the solution in human volunteers, it showed not to be an irritant to the mucosa of the respiratory tree, mouth or the eye tissues. The compound was well tolerated in its aerosol protocol.

The foregoing description conveys the best understanding of the objectives and advantages of the present invention. Different embodiments may be made of the inventive concept of this invention. It's to be understood that all matters disclosed herein are to be interpreted merely as illustrative, and not in a limiting sense.

Summary of the Patent

The Patent is the document confirming an original invention. In this case, the invention is not only the concept of using a solution started from ocean water for the treatment of respiratory diseases, the solution itself. This means the liquid is not just ocean water with algae, sand, plankton and all the matter that form the ocean water, but a combination of ions and elements in the form of a solution with a particular formulation that can be even prepared in a laboratory. The solution can be prepared and bottled for distribution and used in the medical industry or in the form of aerosol. The invention describes different scenarios in how a solution starting from ocean water is used to treat respiratory diseases such as asthma, bronchitis, common colds, and Chronic Obstructive Pulmonary Disease, among others. The solution can serve as a vehicle to deliver substances in the lungs. This means that other medications or substances can be mixed with the solution and once placed in an aerosol machine, the solution can carry the medication to the lungs.

VI) Drinking or Eating Seawater?

Much has been said about the possible benefits of drinking ocean water as a curative therapy. The reality is that no large studies have been conducted to demonstrate the benefit of such a practice. Pictures published at the beginning of the twentieth century showed cases of malnutrition presumably resolved by the use of ocean water as a key component of the diet of the affected patients.

Ocean water contains numerous substances, including minerals and trace elements necessary for a healthy metabolism. The main problem these days is to prepare a formula that does not cause more damage in someone already debilitated. Ocean water is a highly concentrated compound and its consumption may cause diarrhea and further dehydration. One way to use the *good* without the *bad* is obtaining filtered ocean water which still preserves some of the minerals, but in much less concentration. It's called a desalinization process. Through this method, it's possible to make ocean water taste just like regular tap water...even more. Ocean water could be prepared in a way that the new beverage preserves the natural elements. This could add flavor to the drink created. Then, fruit juice, artificial or natural flavor and other nutritious components could be added for the creation of a completely new recipe. A new market could open doors. Imagine tomato juice prepared with natural sea minerals; nutritional formulas comprising the ocean trace elements with a flavor; new pre-packed food to be cooked only with purified ocean water for added flavor and nutritious value. The possibilities are infinite. Prolonged space traveling, submariners, and explorers all over the world could benefit from the new compounds carried on their limited load.

Some companies have given the first steps, but it is needed more from the governments and the research institutions. If we judge for the accidental episodes of swallowing seawater on a vacation by the seashore, it is apparently safe to drink very small amounts of ocean water on regular basis.

However, many questions must be answered before it can be a safe recommendation regarding how much and how frequent one should drink from the ocean. I have heard reports from patients and friends that drinking ocean water, even by accident, can cause loose bowel movements and mild abdominal discomfort. Excessive amounts, as seen in catastrophic conditions at sea, may cause fatal dehydration and brain edema. Research and prudence are the key words.

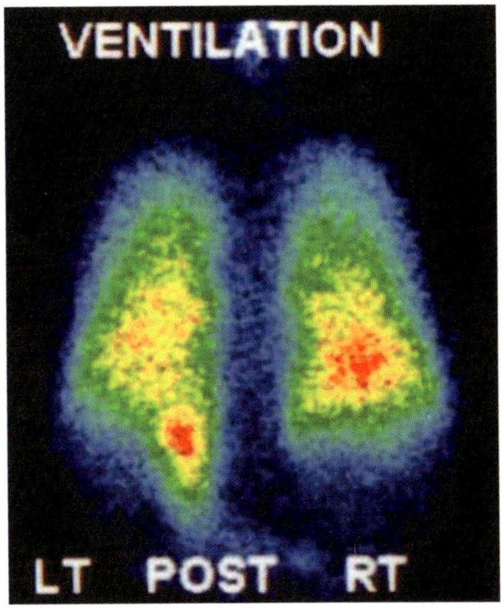

VII) Envisioned Medical Treatments

When I think of the potential uses of ocean water, I think in scientific terms. It has to be critically watched and reevaluated through clinical trials that involve serious statistical tools. Here are some of the principles to follow in seawater therapy when seawater is used as a therapeutic solution. Seawater is without a doubt, the most important element in marine therapy.

Principles of Seawater as a Cosmetic or as a Therapeutic Solution

The following principles are not considered laws, but they should be closely observed when attempting to use seawater for marine therapy beyond its natural sources. One may go to the beach, let's say, to improve psoriatic lesions, and still some principles will be accomplished. These principles don't necessarily have to be present all at once. Some will be accomplished while others might not be present. They are not mutually exclusive, but integrative.

1) ***Seawater therapy must involve the uses of the ocean water mixed with other substances for treatments or as the only therapeutic or cosmetic element used.*** This principle establishes that seawater has to be mixed with other therapeutic elements or as the only marine therapy element.

2) ***Seawater therapy must involve the uses of ocean water during the preparation of the compounds, as part of the formulation or as a vehicle to deliver the compounds***. This refers to the need of the presence of the seawater as part of the preparation of the compounds or the therapy itself.

3) ***Seawater must be used with therapeutic purposes in one or more of the different stages of the matter.*** Depending on the frequency, the administration pathway and

the therapeutic goal, seawater and its minerals **must** be used in a solid form—ice, highly concentrated, or salt contents—in a liquid or semi liquid form (at different concentrations); or in a gaseous stage (in the form of aerosols).

4) ***Seawater must remain purified and sealed.*** For storage and continued use, seawater has to remain protected from accidental contamination since it can carry live elements.

5) ***Seawater must act as a synergistic element during the therapy.*** There is no reason to use seawater as a marine therapy if this compound is not going to enhance the benefits of other cosmetics or therapeutic agents in the process.

6) ***Seawater must remain bio-absorbable after used as a therapeutic agent.*** This principle establishes that seawater is a natural biodegradable product. Seawater should not be transformed during the manufacturing process in a non bioabsorbable matter. Reconstructed seawater might not work in the same form as natural purified ocean water. The cells must be able to absorb and metabolize the elements in their ionic form.

7) ***Seawater must contain minerals or at least trace elements if used for medical or cosmetic purposes.*** The last principle establishes that if marine therapy is the final goal, the purification technology should not go to the point of leaving seawater only in H2O. Minerals and trace elements in the ionic form are the reason to use seawater as a marine therapy. Otherwise, one can use just water.

Marine therapy centers are a future alternative to combine the seawater benefits and the modern technologies and pharmacological advances. A marine therapy center should work ideally as a rehabilitation center and a spa, but always oriented to obtain the medical and cosmetic benefits of seawater. Patients and spa clients in the marine therapy centers would receive the best of both worlds. Many diseases could be treated effectively while changing the body's appearance. They would produce a significant decrease in the length of hospitalization, drug use, and potential side effects of manmade chemicals. A typical user may go on a frequent basis to the center or even stay in a private resort type facility, rather than in the sometimes noisy hospital environment. Still, the person could take the medications, visit her or his doctor, exercise on the water, and enjoy the day at the center. Spas should be more integrated into medical care. They could be a valid alternative for patients needing rehabilitation, early discharge from the hospital, and to treat multiple medical problems happening simultaneously.

When and how to use seawater therapy?

A long list of problems could be included as possible beneficiaries of seawater therapy:

Skin Problems

- Psoriasis
- Atopic dermatitis
- Contact dermatitis
- Eczema
- Actinic Keratosis

- Hyperkeratosis
- Acne

Respiratory Problems

- Sinusitis
- Allergic Rhinitis
- Bronchitis
- Asthma
- Chronic Obstructive Pulmonary Diseases (emphysema, bronchitis asthma)
- Viral respiratory infections
- Atelectasis
- Bronchiectasis

Orthopaedic Problems

- Degenerative Joint Disease
- Rheumatoid Arthritis
- Acute and Chronic Low Back Pain
- Recovery after joints operation or severe injuries

Neurological

- Cerebrovascular accidents and its complications:
- Hemiplegia, monoplegia, paraplegia and sympathetic atrophy

- Nerve paralysis
- Neuromuscular disorders like Muscle dystrophy and Multiple Sclerosis
- Gait disorders

Cardiovascular Problems

- Congestive Heart Failure
- Acute Myocardial Infarction
- Hypertension
- Peripheral vascular Disease

How to use seawater therapy on each particular problem might be the text for a new book. In general, exercising in the water increases the muscle strength. There is almost no impact on the joints. There is better balance and any possible fall is cushioned by the peaceful waters. The ionic minerals may act as the natural skin problem healer and a natural eco system might be the best ally in diseases related to stress, anxiety, and depression. Yes, protocols and research needs to be done in these directions and efforts are already being done in very scattered places around the world. Clinical trials and the support from institutions and governments are definitely needed to open the big doors of medicine to this modality of care. Specific treatments are needed, along with a standard mode of application of the treatments to have measurable results. I am sure there are more benefits to be found after observing the massive use of seawater as a therapeutic modality. Those mentioned in this book are just an illustration.

Let me start by mentioning some of the things that I observed in the laboratory while analyzing the effects of purified ocean water on the human respiratory secretions.

Purified seawater solution (three milliliters) applied in aerosol form using a nebulizer or spray machine for the treatment of nasal congestion, rhinitis or bronchitis. This method would prove the ocean helps to destroy the sticky mucus, bring the phlegm out, and help to decrease the inflammation of the respiratory tract. I have found that purified ocean water destroys the chemical structure of the sputum. The ions present in the natural solution that is the ocean water join the hydrogen bonds separating the water molecules from the phlegm and causing this to dissolve.

Dry phlegm in the respiratory system causes severe dysfunction in persons affected by sinusitis, common colds, bronchitis, emphysema and other common respiratory problems. Have you ever heard people saying that after they went to the beach their cold just got better or went away? It has been well documented that there is improvement of the nasal symptoms after using purified ocean water.

Another scientific breakthrough has been the combination of purified ocean water and steroids (***seanolone***) or seawater and a bronchodilator (***seabuterol***) which could be excellent not only for skin problems (only ***seanolone***), but both can be an extraordinary addition for the management of asthma, Chronic Obstructive Pulmonary Disease and many other respiratory problems. I have prepared formulations that can be applied in the form of aerosol. The combination of medications like those used in asthma, the steroids and bronchodilators, with ocean water purified by my method, does not produce any crystallization of the elements and allows their application by aerosol methods.

This could open a door to a new class of medications. Seawater is not a simple vehicle. It's a very active compound that interacts with other substances that then form new compounds with better effects in the human body.

The need for clinical trials is imperative. Humankind is waiting for the big pharmaceutical companies to overcome the fear of duplication of their products as a driving force to decide what is going to the research and development pipelines and then to the production lines. There are so many people in need. They can be counted for hundreds of millions all over the world.

VIII) A New Discovery

The last paragraph of the patent was prophetic in reality. I decided to prove in a tangible way that the solution was an extraordinary vehicle for medications and there was no better way to do so than attempting to use a radionuclide commonly used as a diagnostic method of pulmonary problems in medical centers.

The solution proved to be an excellent vehicle for radioactive substances for diagnostic radiological procedures. A ventilation scan study was done using technetium 99m, mixed directly with ocean water and given to a subject (in this case, the investigator himself) through an aerosol device. Technetium 99m is a form of radioactive Technetium, which is used safely in the medical industry to discover serious pulmonary clots or problems, and to indicate a mismatch between the air breathed and the blood available in the lungs. The test concluded that the solution was able to carry the radionuclide to the human lungs without any complication, and it could produce similar radiological images than those observed with a more costly traditional premixing of the radionuclide with colloids.

The experience proved the distribution of the ocean water solution in the human lungs. It demonstrated a perfect tolerability of the compound and it proved not only that it is feasible and safe, but that it can be used as a vehicle. I took the test like any other patient. The gamma camera was calibrated first. Then the solution was mixed directly with the radioactive substance and I received the aerosol with the material. Obviously, a step has been skipped. Normally, as part of the protocol, the radioactive material is mixed first with a colloid type of substance that allows its transport activated to the lungs. This time, the colloid was not used and a new discovery happened.

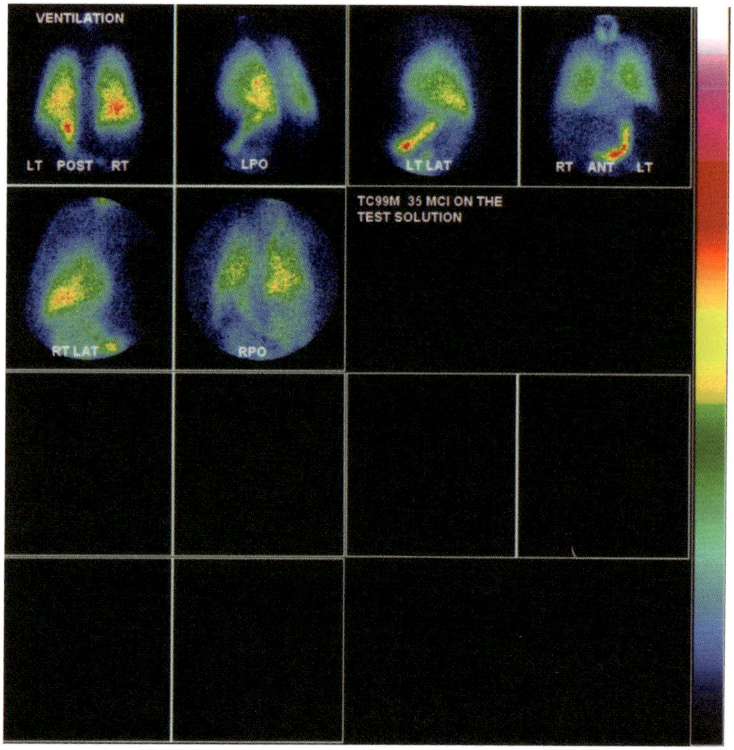

The experiment showed not only the feasibility to take substances to the human lungs, but the capacity of the compound to bind through its ions complex compounds and in this particular case, radioactive materials without altering its properties and functions. This opens new doors in medicine for the possible use of the compound for medical radio diagnostic procedures. My appreciation to Dr. Rauven Porges, M.D., Chief of Radiologyof Sheridan Healthcare Corporation and Consultant for this experiment. Dr. Porges was very instrumental in the preparation of the conditions for the experimental protocol and the facilitation of the necessary equipment, staff and materials for testing.

How Does the Ocean Clean Our Lungs? The Mechanism of Action

What originally sparked my scientific interest in the ocean was to find out if the sea truly can help us to breathe better or if this was just another myth about the seas. I always need to find proof; something that will really convince the doctors around the world of the benefits and the need to incorporate this modality of care in our armamentarium to treat diseases. Seawater properly prepared makes patients feel better and probably helps them to heal faster. The effect of a treatment with purified ocean water might simply be staying healthier for longer periods of time.

What follows is an explanation of a scientific experiment dedicated to observe what a solution obtained from ocean water can do to human respiratory secretions.

The scientific community wants facts. I need them to either abandon unnecessary efforts, and the costs involved on a patent development, or pursue a scientific passion. I decided to test the solution in the laboratory and this is what happened.

Once the solution was prepared, I used an aerosol machine to apply the seawater over human respiratory secretions. After about ten minutes of application via the aerosol, the thick phlegm became very liquid, less adhesive, and started melting down. That's exactly what happens when we go to the beach while having a common cold. We suddenly start breathing better, and all the phlegm starts to clear.

I took the glass slides with the test results to a pathologist, Dr. Kip Amazon. He reviewed them and noticed that the solution did not cause any toxic effect over the human cells. They were intact. The microscopic study also showed me that the phlegm shape changed once given an aerosol and that the protein that forms the human phlegm, named mucin, is transformed under the effect of the ions of the solution. I thought this would be crucial for patients affected by asthma, bronchitis, common colds, sinusitis, emphysema, and other respiratory problems. That's why the secretions become liquid, and can be easily expelled from the lungs or the sinuses when we go to the beach! This is called an expectorant effect and the mechanism is a protein cleavage. I had just found something, until then, unpublished. I decided that the medical community needed to know about these findings immediately. The following report was sent to The Journal of Aerosol Medicine, in New York City. Because of the current preparation of the book, we decided not to respond to the panel that evaluated the article for its publication. The article was registered with the Library of Congress in Washington, D.C. and is written in a language more appropriate for healthcare professionals rather than a general public. I decided to include it in this book as medical literature has always been a subject of discrete research by the general public which loves to see sometimes what doctors have to say to other doctors. I hope you enjoy it.

Summary of the article:

Once an investigator makes a discovery, either small or big, an article should be written as a form of immediate communication to the scientific community about the findings. The present article narrates the initial findings of how the solution acts on human sputum (phlegm) and possibly helps to clean the human respiratory tract. The communication was submitted to the Journal of Aerosol Medicine. After reviewing the journal's expert critique, the author decided not to transfer the rights for publication considering its possible inclusion in this book. The article has not being changed and narrates the original way the discovery was made. It describes the action of the solution on human phlegm and the way this was observed. It details the method followed to prove the effects of purified ocean water in the human secretions and how this could impact the health of many people all over the world. The article discusses how the compound makes its effects and explains the need for clinical trials as well as future uses of the solution as a vehicle for other substances.

ORIGINAL SCIENTIFIC ARTICLE

EFFECTS OF A SOLUTION COMPRISING SEA WATER ON HUMAN SPUTUM.

INTRODUCTION

Secretions from the upper and lower respiratory tract become very viscous during inflammatory states. Upper respiratory infections, asthma, acute bronchitis, chronic obstructive pulmonary disease, and cystic fibrosis are among the problems where more commonly accumulation of respiratory secretions causes an additional burden to the patients (1) (2) (6). When the sputum becomes dry, the normal gas exchange is altered and the mucus plugs resulting may lead to a significant worsening in the pulmonary function. This eventually leads to cardio-respiratory arrest or serious pulmonary complications.

Expectorants and mucolytics have been used in the past to treat acute and chronic respiratory conditions mostly in the form of pills or syrups. Sodium Chloride at 0.9 percent in an aerosol form helps remove secretions; however, lack of credibility by doctors and patients might be limiting its current use. Other expectorants have failed to prove efficacy or associated side effects such as palpitations or blood pressure elevation creating a compliance challenge (5). Inhaled substances like Acetylcysteine have side effects that are unacceptable for many patients. Sterile seawater sprays have shown to improve symptoms of rhinitis (4).

The frequent observation of patients affected with common colds and/or sinusitis that report improvement in their conditions as an effect of a seawater bath has made us to test a solution starting from raw ocean water to evaluate its effect on human sputum. The new compound was subjected to a purification process to prove its properties as mucolytic and possibly as expectorant. Other compounds starting from seawater are currently used to produce a mechanical *lavage* of the nostrils in rhinitis (7).

MATERIALS AND METHOD

Seawater was collected from the Atlantic Ocean at 1.7 nautical miles from the shores of Bal Harbor in the area of Miami, Florida. The zone is influenced by the Gulf Stream. Ocean water was obtained from seventeen feet of depth, beyond the plankton habitat and any possible surface contaminant. A decantation process was performed using a one micron carbon activated, micro filter model Pur FM 3000, lot code 3310422302 and manufactured by PUR Water Purification Products, Inc., Minneapolis, Minnesota, United States of America. The filter was used to remove residual plankton or marine life and to reduce to minimum potential contaminants such as mercury, benzene, carbofuran, and lead. The resulting compound was composed by six elements considered the active ingredients and present in the form of totally dissolved salts or isolated ions. Composition of the solution was double checked by three laboratory analyses to test the consistency of the results using the standard technique and equipment available to test urine electrolytes. Although there are more than sixty different trace elements in ocean water, these were not quantified for the experiment. The most common ions in the solution were chloride (also, the most abundant in the human body), sodium, magnesium, sulfate, potassium and calcium. The formation of pharmacologically active salts was not measured. No precipitates were present at any moment during the experiment. After tested in the laboratory, the solution obtained was identical to that marketed as Sea-Mar® by SeaMyst Corporation of Miami Beach, Florida.

Two slides containing the sputum from the lower respiratory tract of a volunteer affected by acute bronchitis were placed at a thirty degree angle to quantify their descent at a room temperature of seventy-two degrees, and a relative humidity of 78 percent. The slides with sputum were marked indicating the sputum extension, 30 millimeters (± 2.5) and left to rest at thirty degrees. The sputum descent was quantified and measured until the sputum stopped the descend process and a steady state was reached at fifteen minutes. The slides were marked again at 38 millimeters (± 3.5) and this was considered the starting point to measure the sputum descend under the aerosol effect. After zeroing the sputum starting point, the slides were subjected to a nebulization of 3 milliliters of the solution during ten minutes each. The volunteer provided the sputum samples right before the experiment and was taking only acetaminophen for symptoms at the time of the specimen collection. The aerosol machine mouthpiece was located at twelve inches from the slides to avoid a direct impact of the aerosol stream. Two control slides contained sputum from the lower respiratory tract from the same individual, and were equally positioned at a thirty-degree angle, away from the nebulization area; and did not receive any treatment (non treatment group). The experience was repeated on two more occasions separated by a period of twenty-four hours in the same week using a conventional aerosol machine Voyage II, model 277, manufactured in Italy and distributed by Mada Medical Products, Inc. Six slides went under treatment and six were used as a control group. Immediately after the aerosol treatment was concluded, the slides were fixed in a formalin solution and later colored with hematoxiline and eosin for pathology analysis.

RESULTS

It was proved that a solution created from ocean water can be delivered via aerosol in the form of a steady stream of micro-drops using a conventional aerosol machine. The solution changed the rheological properties of the sputum. There were no cytological changes. The respiratory tract cells in the sputum and bacteria isolated or forming chains were still identifiable after the aerosol treatment.

MACROSCOPIC OBSERVATIONS

The viscosity of the sputum receiving the aerosol decreased making the sputum less viscous and transparent and causing the secretions to slide down through the microscope glass previously positioned at a thirty-degree angle. The total volume displacement of the secretion was 6 millimeters (± 2.5, mode 6) representing 15.78 percent of volume variation after receiving the aerosol. The displacement of the sputum that did not receive the aerosol compound was 0.5 millimeters (± 0.5, mode 0.5) representing a 1.31 percent displacement of the sputum over the slide. The mean of the sputum descent was 9.75. The mode was 3.25. The volume displaced in the sputum treated with an aerosol was twelve times bigger than those not treated. No crystal accumulations or precipitations were observed on the slides treated with the aerosolized compound. A residual liquid was formed right below the sputum receiving the aerosol and it was not measured as part of the sputum descent.

MICROSCOPIC OBSERVATIONS

No cytological changes were observed and no crystal deposits were found. Bacteria and cellular morphology remained intact and identifiable. A change in the shape and consistency of the sputum receiving the aerosolized compound was observed. Sputum not receiving the aerosol maintained a linear pattern of mucin.

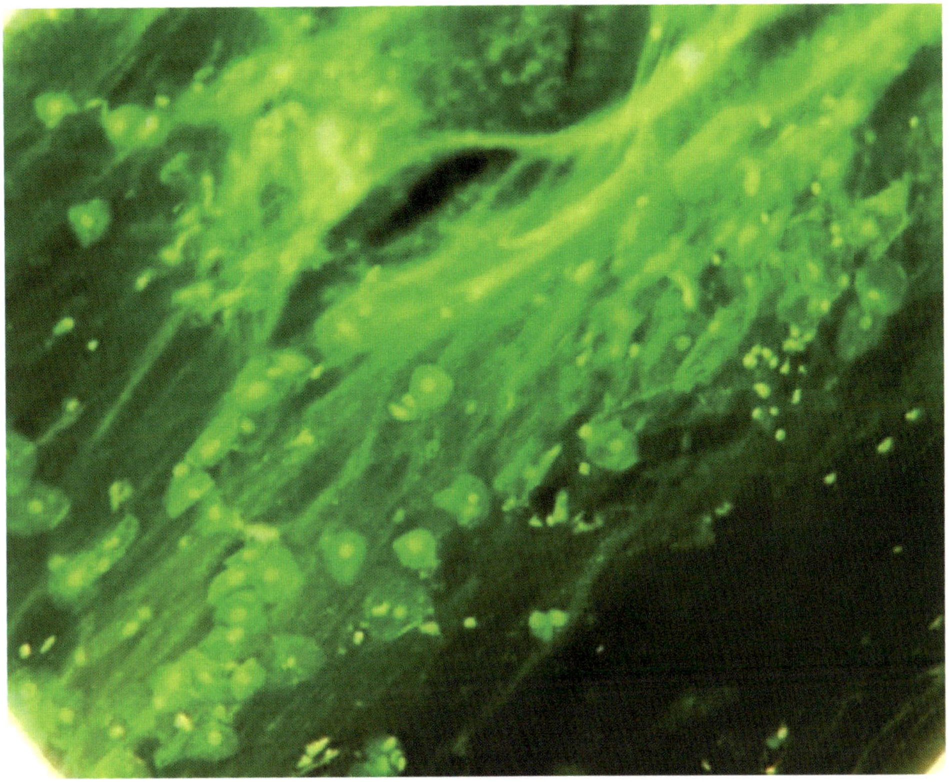

(illustration 1) while the sputum receiving the treatment showed a circular sponge-like pattern and more liquid filled spaces in all the slides treated with the nebulized solution.

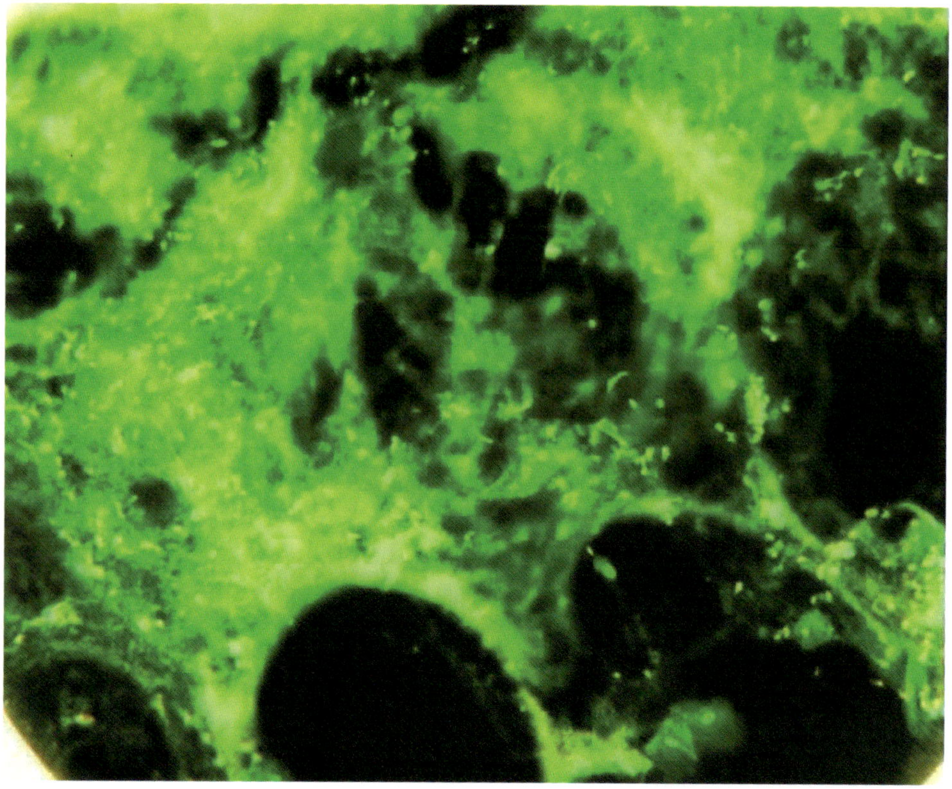

(illustration 2) It was observed that less cells in the slides were subjected to the aerosol solution.

DISCUSSION

The changes observed in the rheological properties of the sputum from the lower respiratory tract after exposed to an aerosol solution obtained from ocean water were not previously published and might have several implications. First, this model could validate the observation of patients affected by respiratory infections that reported a significant improvement following a day on the beach. The retraction observed in the mucin pattern and the attraction of more liquid into the sputum structure that made the secretions less viscous suggests that the solution may have an expectorant effect in mammals since these phenomena might make the sputum easier to expel from the respiratory structures. The compound activity on the secretions suggests a change in the surface tension of the sputum, because of the interaction with the mix of salts dissolved in the ocean water, particularly sodium, magnesium, calcium, and potassium which were positively charged ions. It is suggested that the Mechanism of Action is a protein cleavage of the mucin explained by the bonds of the solution cations to the negatively charged Sialic acid molecules. In addition to this, hydrogen bonds present in the mucin were broken allowing the formation of new chemical bonds with chloride and sulfate present in the solution—all of which leads to a chemical cleavage of the mucin structure. These phenomena could be explained given that the salts are composed by pharmacologically active elements (not crystals) in the form of totally dissolved solids and the ionic chemical bonds between the salts allow chemical interactions with other substances. The changes in the surface tensions of the phlegm may cause a progressive reshape of the secretions of the respiratory tract of mammals that would allow the mechanisms for the expulsion of the phlegm being more effective. This rearrangement of the tension forces and the action of the salts may cause the transformation to be a more liquid type of fluid and the downward displacement of secretion observed on the slides.

The pathological observations that the solution did not affect the cellular structures would allow further microscopic analysis in clinical grounds on sputum from presumptively treated patients and still making feasible morphological diagnosis. The same principle applies for pathological organisms observed in the sputum in case of the need for microbiological identification. The smaller cell count in the slides subjected to the aerosolized solution may respond to the *lavage* effect of the compound dragging down the cells present in the sputum by a gravity effect.

Other important considerations are that the solution has no artificial ingredients and it contains trace elements, which may play a role if the compound is given as a treatment to mammals on a regular basis. Zinc is a cofactor necessary for the action of Carbonic Anhydrase during the conversion of $CO_2 + H_2O$ into $HCO_3 + H^+$ and salts as Magnesium Sulfate and calcium may play a role activating the Second Messenger mechanism and causing bronchial muscle relaxation. The six key elements of the solution maintains almost a sequent position in the Mendeleyev Periodic Table—Sodium 11, Magnesium 12, Sulfur 16, Chloride 17, Potassium 18, and Calcium 19. This particular disposition of the key elements paired in three groups is unique in earth and it is believed that by duplicating the characteristics and chemical properties of each element the compound is much more stable. Another grouping distribution of the compound is the association of the four cations—sodium, potassium, calcium and magnesium as metals and the two anions sulfur and chloride as non metals.

The fact that the solution is hypertonic may help to trigger an osmotic mechanism through the membrane of the Goblets cells making the sputum even more humid. The compound showed no signs of cytotoxicity, which could make it an excellent delivery vehicle for biotechnological products and medications, which might exhibit a synergistic effect.

Its cost effectiveness could make the treatments reachable to a broader population sector. More studies could address if there is in fact cellular preservation since there were no cytological changes observed which could represent a sign of membrane stabilization, which could have an implication in the treatment of asthma and allergic rhinitis.

Although more studies need to be made using a broader number of slides and animal models, the protocol is reproducible and the results are constant. These open opportunities for further studies use a solution starting from seawater in a sterile form in human subjects as an expectorant, mucolytic and possibly as a decongestant to treat conditions such as common colds and acute sinusitis. Furthermore, the compound has the potential to become an ideal vehicle to deliver other drugs in the respiratory system considering its safety and the capacity to make the secretions more liquid, which could facilitate the penetration of therapeutic drugs into deeper pulmonary structures.

AKNOWLEDGMENTS

I appreciated the effort of Kip Amazon, M.D., and Victor Ramirez, M.D. from

Aventura, Florida for the pathology analysis of the slides. I want to thank Carlos Santos, M.D. Pulmonologist, for the evaluation and review of the experimental results and his valuable input.

REFERENCES

1. Del Mar, C., and Glasziou, P. 2003. Upper Respiratory Tract Infection. In Clinical Evidence Concise. Ed. BMJ Publishing Group, London. 326-327.
2. Taccariello, M., Parikh A., Darby Y., and Scadding, G. 1999. Nasal Douching as a Valuable Adjunct in The Management of Chronic Rhinosinusitis. Rhinology. 37: 29-32.
3. Harari, M., Barzillai, R., and Shani, J. 1998. Magnesium In The Management Of Asthma: Critical Review of Acute and Chronic Treatment, and Deutsches Medizinisches Zentrum's (DMZ) clinical experience at the Dead Sea. J. Asthma. 35: 525-536.
4. Bousquet, J., Cauwenberge, P.V., Khaltaev, N., and Allergic Rhinitis and its Impact on Asthma (ARIA) Workshop Group-Independent Expert Panel. 2001. Allergic Rhinitis and its Impact on Asthma. J. Allergy Clin. Immunol. 108:S147-334.
5. Allen, G., Kelsberg, G., and Jankowski, T.A. 2003. Do Nasal Decongestants Relieve Symptoms? The Journal of Family Practice. 8:721-722
6. Fiel, S., Kane, G.C., and Petty, T.L. 2002. Evaluating and treating chronic cough. Patient Care. 14:29-39.
7. Papsin, B., and Mctavish, A. 2003. Saline Nasal Irrigation Its Role as an Adjunct Treatment. Can. Fam. Physician 49: 168-173.

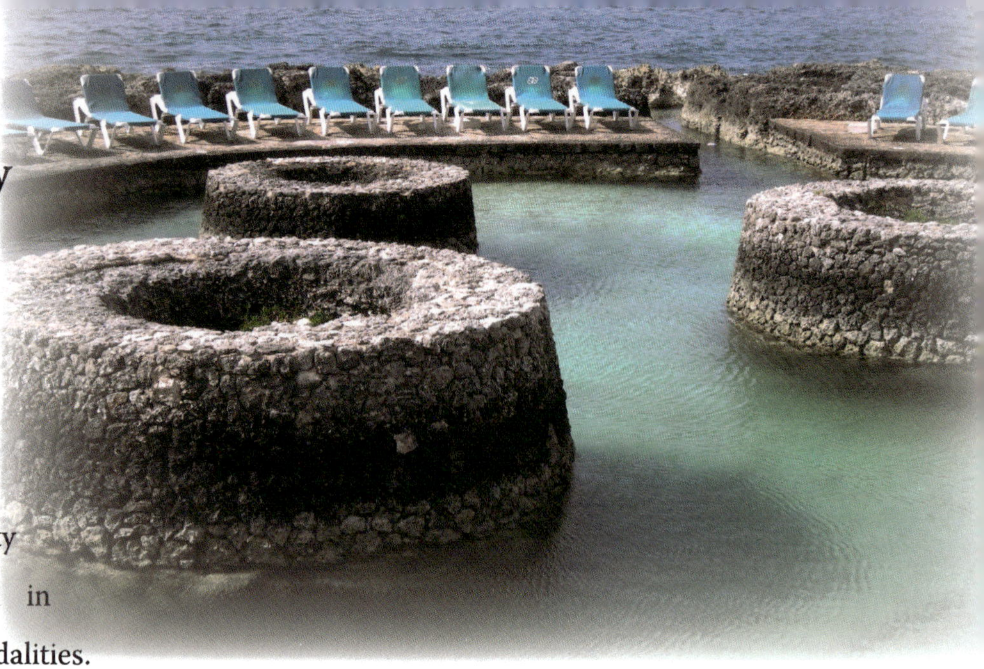

Marine Therapy Centers and Services around the World

There is an increasing interest by the hospitality industry around the world in providing marine therapy modalities. It might be in the form of spa procedures or just centers dedicated to the treatment of patients and clients seeking nonmedical modalities of treatment. The centers offer a variety of services, but some of these services must be coordinated ahead of time. There is no special recommendation or preference for any center. This is just a mere compilation of information to serve the traveling reader. The contact information sometimes includes the e-mail and web site URL. I strongly recommend that all travelers call the facilities directly or speak with your travel advisor prior to any ticketing. Make sure the facilities are operational and are not going through repairs or remodeling while you are on your vacation. Always ask if they offer particular services that you might be expecting. You may find it interesting to search on the Internet before traveling to places. It can really give you a deeper insight of what to expect and even to read reports from people who have already visited the places listed. The following list might be a good lead to your personal search.

Argentina

Aquae Sulis
Independencia 250 (7240)
Lobos – Buenos Aires –
Argentina 02227 - 42 3940 / 42 4330 / 42 1931
INFORMES Y RESERVAS
Telephone/Fax: (54) (011) 4 658 - 1226 / 8218
E-mail: aquaeinfo@aquaesulis.com.ar www.aquaesulis.com.ar

Canada

Auberge du Parc de Paspebiac
Auberge Du Parc INN 68,
Gérard D. Lévesque O. C.P.40, Paspébiac, Qc
G0C 2K0 CANADA
Telephone: 1-800-463-0890
Fax: 1-418-752-6406
abp@aubergeduparc.com

Kingsbrae Arms. St Andrews by the Sea
219 King Street
St. Andrews, New Brunswick
ESB 1y1 Canada
Telephone: 506 529 1897
www.kingsbrae.com

Chile

Puyuhuapi Lodge and Spa
Bahia Dorita s/n
Puyuhuapi. Chile
Telephone/fax (56-57) 325103/ 325117/325129
www.patagonia-connection.com

The Radisson Acqua Hotel and Spa Concón (near Viña del Mar)
Conco, CL
Av. Borgono 23333
Concon. Chile
www.hotels.com

France

Hôtel Best Western Thalasstonic
Douarnenez - Finistère (29) - Bretagne - France
Informations et Réservations Tel. 00 33 2 98744747

Novotel Thalassa Dinard
Dinard - Ille-et-Vilaine (35) - Bretagne - France
Informations et Réservations Tel. 00 33 2 99167810

Sofitel Thalassa Quiberon
Quiberon - Morbihan (56) - Bretagne - France
Informations et Réservations Tel. 00 33 (0)2 97502000

Hôtel Ti Al Lannec
Trébeurden - Côtes-D'Armor (22) - Bretagne - France
Informations et Réservations Tel. 00 33 2 96 15 01 01

\Le Grand Hôtel Des Thermes
Saint-Malo - Ille-et-Vilaine (35) - Bretagne - France
Informations et Réservations Tel. 00 33 (0)2 99 40 75 00

Hotel Antinea
Saint-Malo - Ille-et-Vilaine (35) - Bretagne - France
Informations et Réservations Tel. +33 (0)2 99 56 10 75

Mercure Thalassa Les Sables d'Olonne
Lac de Tanchet 85100 Les Sables d'Olonne - France
Telephone: (+33) 2/51217777 Fax (+33) 2/51217780
www.mercure.com

French Polynesia

Intercontinental Bora Bora Resort & Thalasso Spa
BP 156
Bora Bora, 98730 French Polynesia
Telephone: (689) 607600
Fax: (689) 607699
www.boraboraspa.interconti.com

Greece

Blue Palace Resort & Spa. The Elounda Spa & Thalassotherapy
P.O. Box 38 Elounda
Crete, Greece 720 53
Telephone: 30 - 28410 – 65500

Italy

Hotel Marinedda Thalasso & Spa
Isola Rossa - Portobello -
Sassari - Sardegna - Italia Numero Verde
Telephone: 199.720.693

Sofitel Thalassa Timi Ama
Località Notteri - Villasimius -
Cagliari - Sardegna - Italia
Telephone: 199.720.693

Mexico

Paraiso de la Bonita Resort & Thalasso
Carretera Chetumal-Cancun, Km 328, SM 31,
Bahia Petempich, Puerto Morelos, Q. Roo, Mexico 77580

Telephone: +52 (998) 872 8300
Fax: +52 (998) 872 8301

Playa Grande Thalasso Spa
Avenida Playa Grande #1, Cabo San Lucas, BCS Mexico
Open daily: 8:00 a.m. to 8:00 p.m.
Telephone: (624) 143-7575

Occidental Grand Xcaret
Carretera Federal Chetumal-Puerto Juarez Km 282
307
77710 Solidaridad Quintana Roo, Mexico
Telephone 866-324-7795 or 52-984-871-5400
www.occidentalhotels.com

Polynesia

Intercontinental Bora Bora Resort & Thalasso Spa
BP 156
Bora Bora, 98730 French Polynesia
Telephone: (689) 607600
Fax: (689) 607699
www.boraboraspa.interconti.com

Russia

Golden Ring Hotel
5Smolenskaya Street
Moscow, Russia
119121
www.hotel-rates.com

Spain

Dunas La Canaria

C/ Barranco de la Verga, s/n - Arguineguín-Gran Canaria -

Las Palmas - Islas Canarias - España
Information and Reservations Telephone + 34 928 150 400
Hotel Byblos Andaluz

Urb. Mijas Golf - Mijas Costa -
Málaga - Andalucía - España
Telephone: + 34 952 473050

Gran Tacande Hotel & Spa
c/ Alcalde Walter Paetzmann s/n - Costa Adeje-Tenerife -
Sta. Cruz Tenerife - Islas Canarias - España
Telephone: + 34 922 746400

Hotel Gloria Palace Amadores
C/ La Palma, 2 - Mogán-Gran Canaria -
Las Palmas - Islas Canarias - España
Telephone: + 34 928 128510
Hotel Cleopatra Palace

Av. de las Américas s/n - Playa de las Américas-Tenerife -
Sta. Cruz Tenerife - Islas Canarias - España
Telephone: + 34 922 757545

United Kingdom

La Joie de Vivre
75 - 77 High Street
High Street
Cranleigh
Surrey
GU6 8AU
Telephone: 01483 272379

Fax: 01483 267083
sales@lajoiedevivre.co.uk

United States of America

Fort Lauderdale

Hyatt Regency Pier 66
2301 S.E. 17th Street
Fort Lauderdale, FL 33316 USA
Telephone: 954 525 6666
Fax: 954 728 3541

Key West

Pier House
One Duval Street
Key West, FL 33040 USA
Telephone: 305-296-4600, 800-723-2791
Fax: 305-296-7569
E-mail the hotel: mailto:info@pierhouse.com

Miami

Dezerland Hotel
Nirvana Spa
8701 Collins Avenue
Miami Beach, FL 33154
Telephone: 305-867-4850
Fax: 305-867-8126

Mandarin Oriental
500 Brickell Key Drive
Miami, FL 33131
Telephone: 305-913-8288
Fax: 305-913-8300

E-mail:momia-reservations@mohg.com
Web site: www.mandarinoriental.com

The Ritz-Carlton
455 Grand Bay Dr.
Key Biscayne, FL 33149
Telephone: 305-365-4500
Fax: 305-365-4505

Fairmont Turnberry Isle Resort & Club
19999 W. Country Club Drive,
Aventura, FL 33180-2401 USA
Telephone: 305-932-6200
Fax: 305- 932-6560

Acqualina Resort & Spa
17875 Collins Ave.
Sunny Isles Beach, FL 33160
Telephone: 305-918-8000 or 888-804-4338
Fax: 305-918-8100
E-mail: reservations@acqualina.com

Double Tree Ocean Point Resort and Spa
17375 Collins Avenue
Sunny Isles Beach, FL 33160
Toll-free: 866-623-2678
Fax: 786-528-2519

New York

Gurneys-Inn Spa and Resort
290 Old Montauk Highway

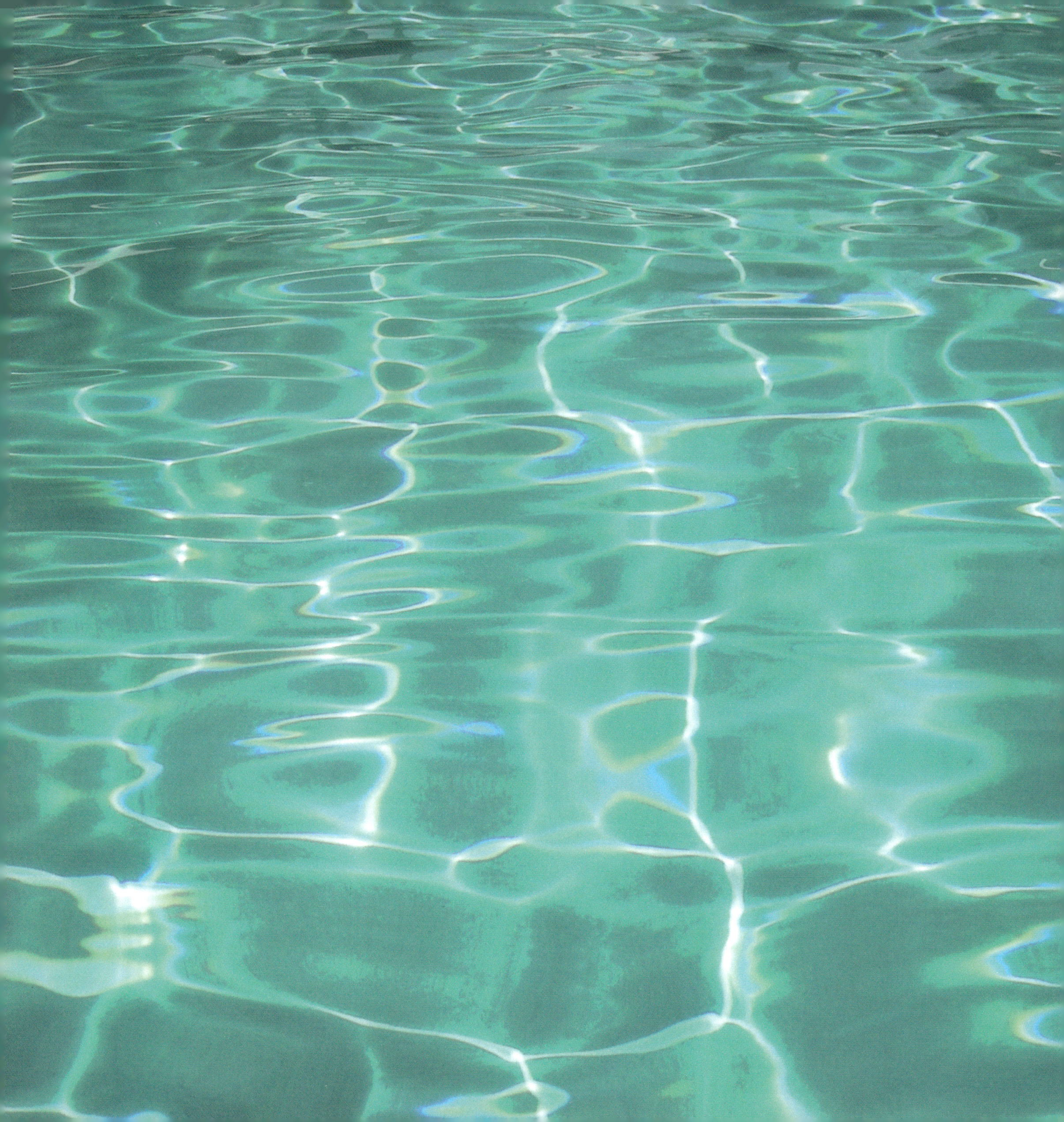

She is kind and very beautiful. He always thought of the sea as *la mar* which is what people call her in Spanish when they love her.

—Ernest Hemingway, *The Old Man and the Sea*, 1952.

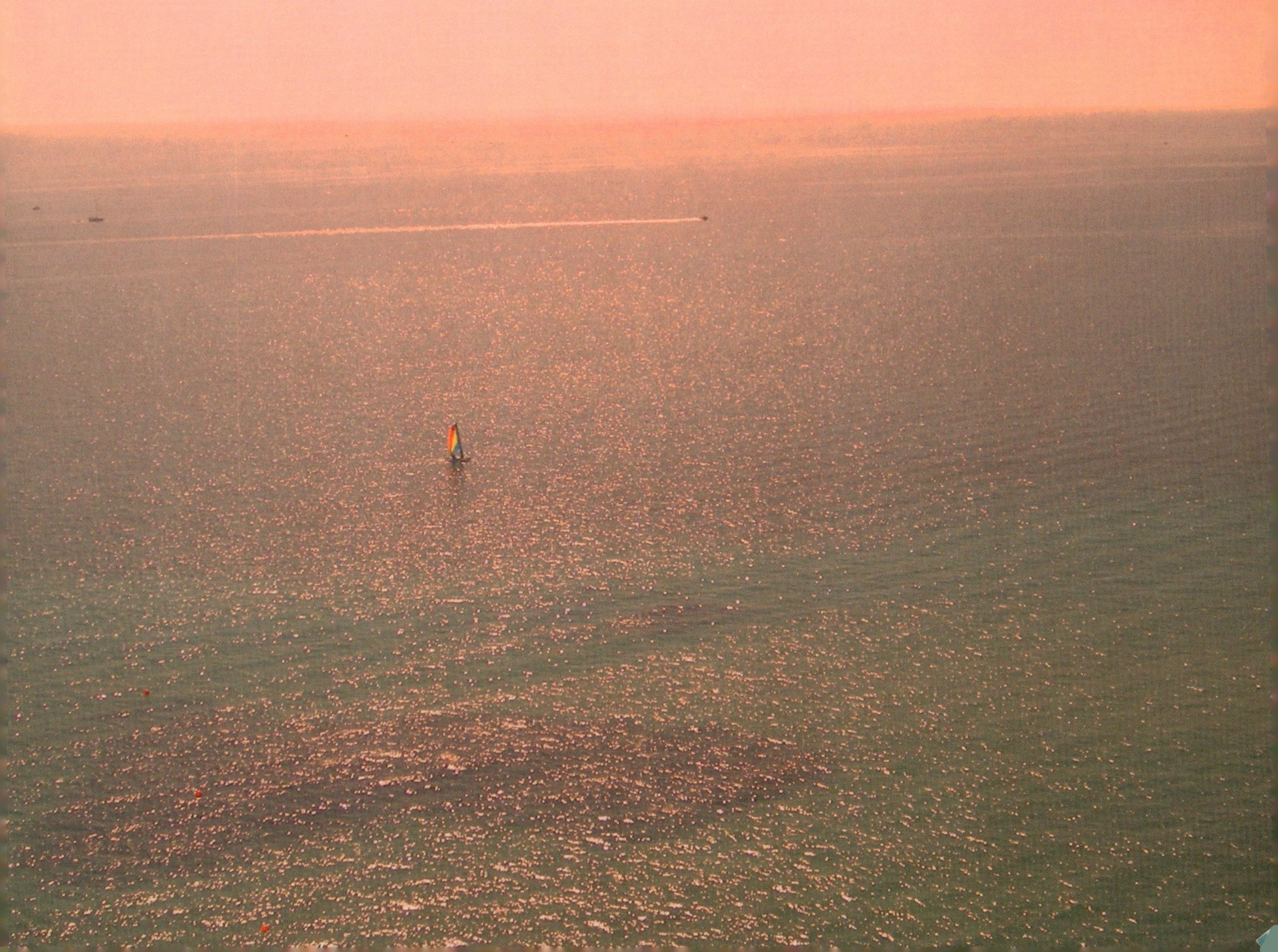

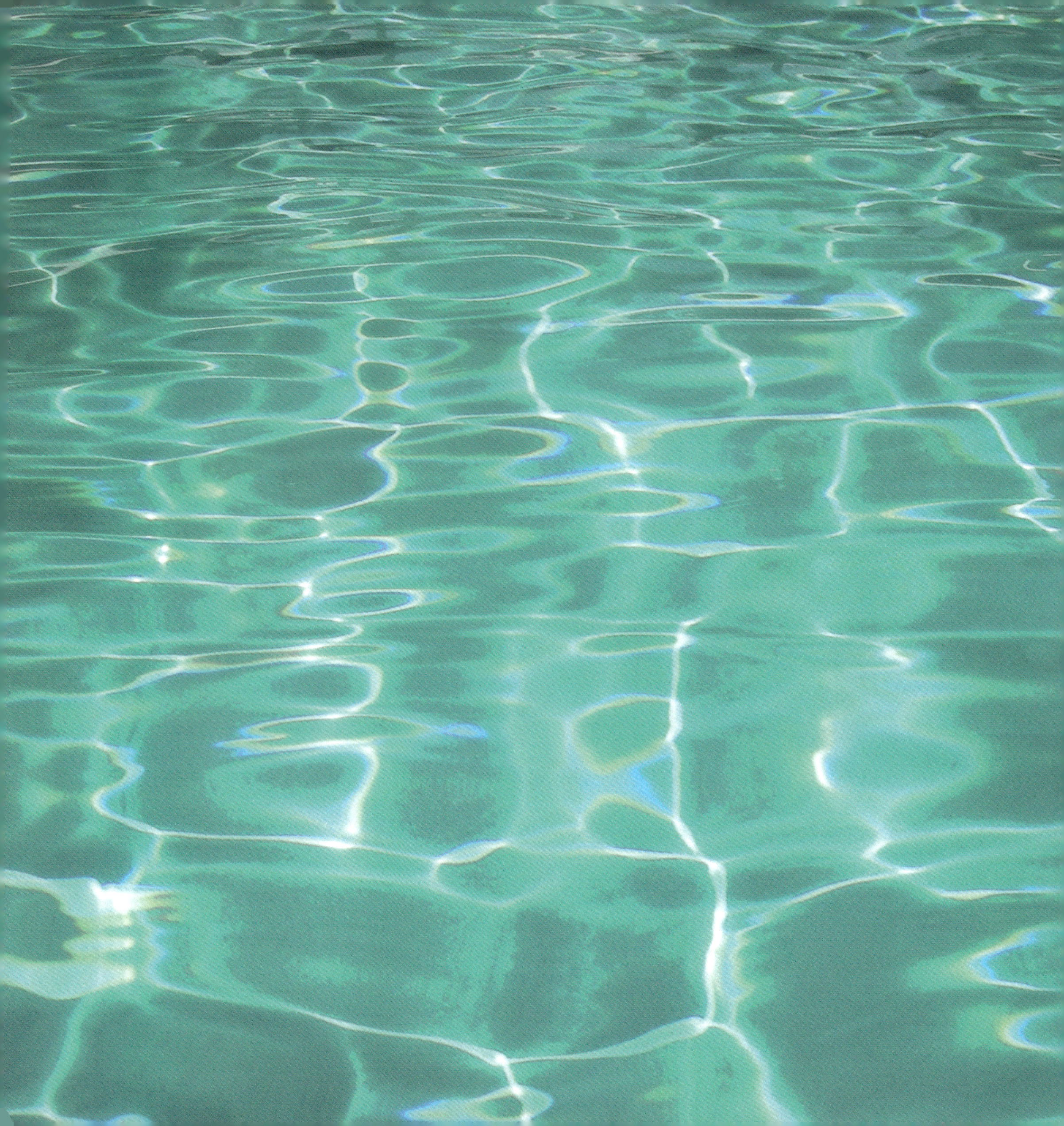

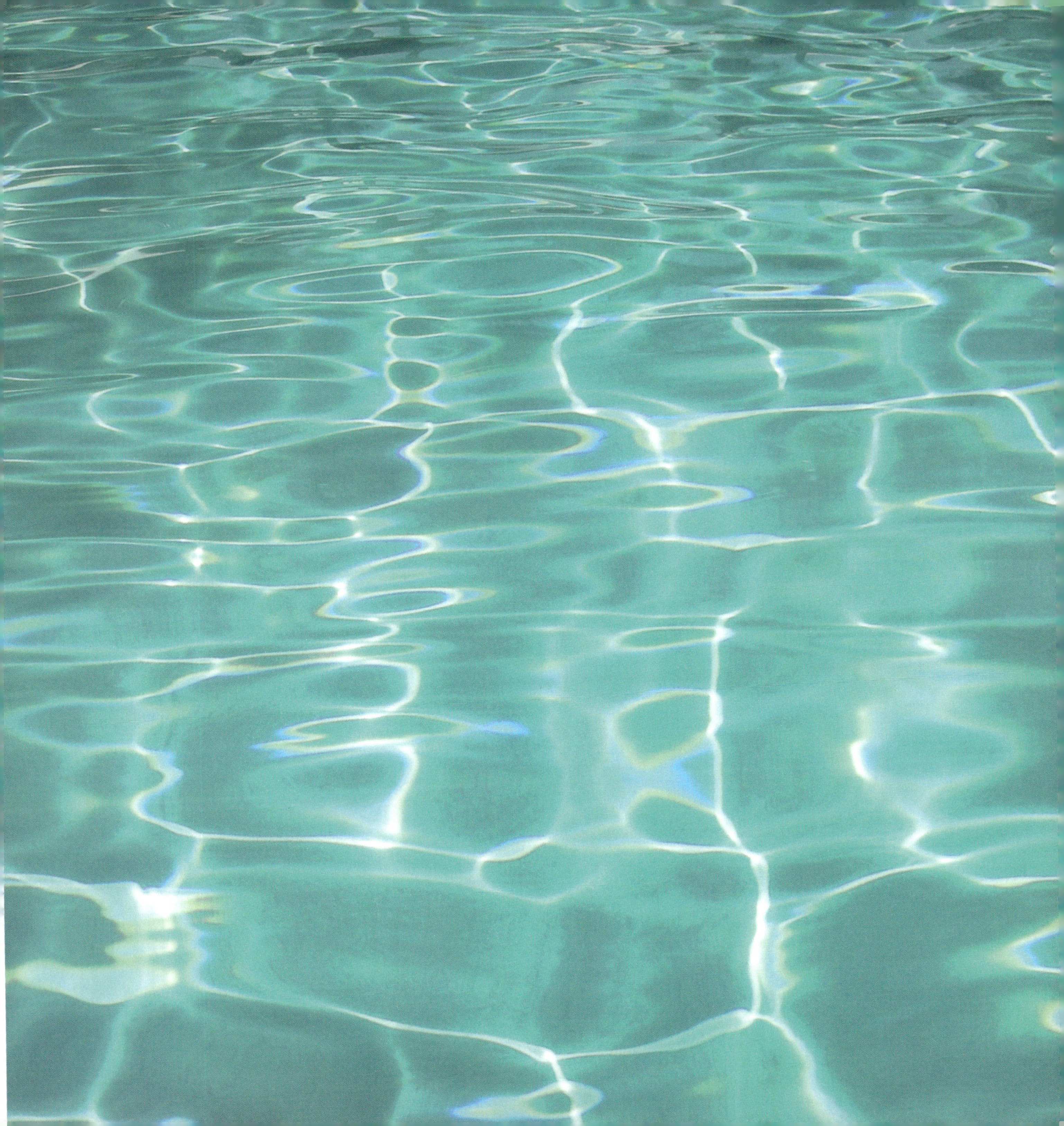

LaVergne, TN USA
01 November 2010
2014LVUK00002B

FRAG doch mal ...

Sylvia Englert

Sterne und Planeten

Mit Illustrationen von
Johann Brandstetter

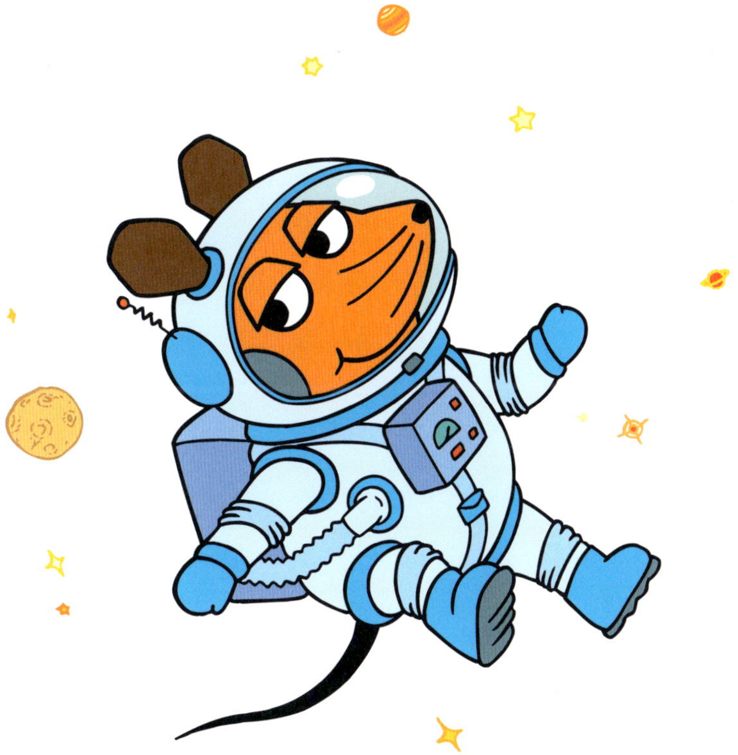

CARLSEN

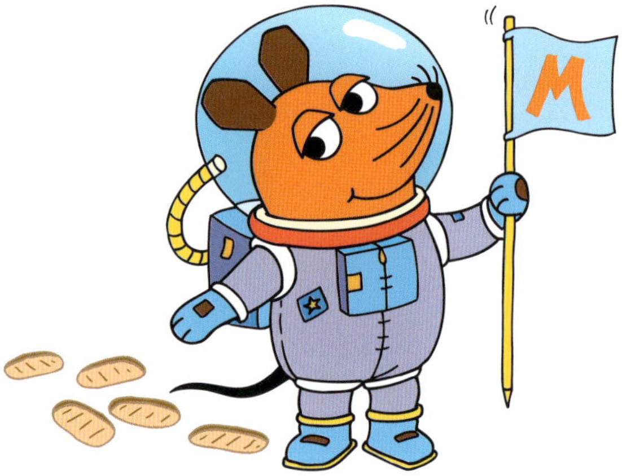

MIX
Papier aus verantwortungsvollen Quellen
FSC® C018236
www.fsc.org

Texte: Sylvia Englert
Illustrationen: Johann Brandstetter
Mausillustrationen: Ina Mertens
Frag doch mal-Logo: Udo Schöbel
Umschlagbild: Fotolia © Vadimsadovski
Bildnachweis für Innenfotos: Fotolia: 11 (3dsculptor), 14 (Grafvision), 19 (alexlmx), 23 (viechie81), 29 (Peter Kirschner), 33 (aapsky), 42 (Joshua Resnick), 44 (passmil198216), 46 (Jürgen Fälchle), 47 (3dsculptor);
GettyImages, München: 31 o. (Roger Ressmeyer); Mauritius Images, Mittenwald: 53 (AGE Fotostock);
NASA: 9, 51; NASA/JPL-Caltech: 5, 24, 25 (Courtesy/JPL-Caltech), 38;
Picture-alliance, Frankfurt/M.: 33 (dpa), 52 (dpa); Pixabay (PD): 4 (WikiImages);
Shutterstock: 31 u. (jorisvo)
Lektorat: Christine Mildner
Redaktion: Katharina Eisele
Gestaltung und Satz: awendrich grafix, Hamburg
ISBN 978-3-551-25243-2
www.carlsen.de

Inhalt

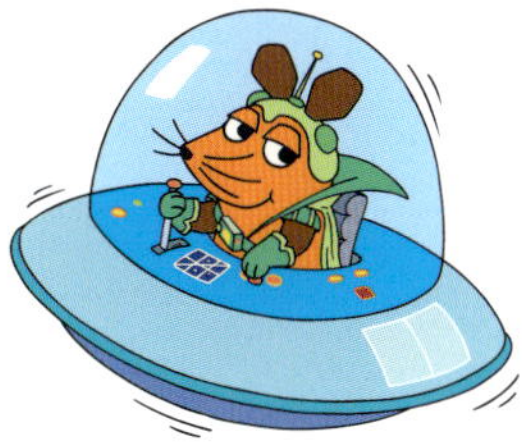

Ist die Erde wirklich rund?

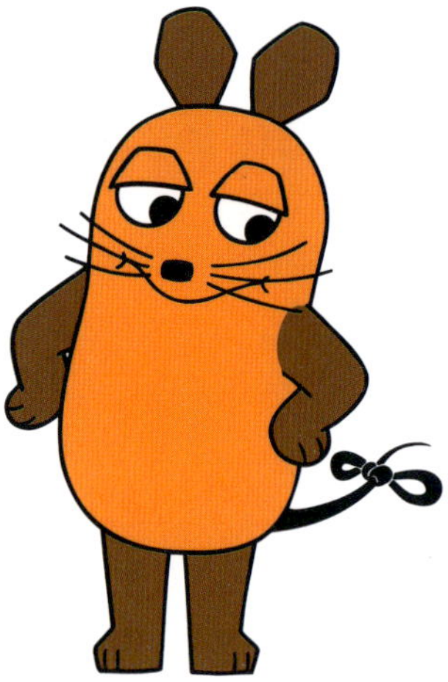

Normalerweise kann man nicht sehen, dass die Erde eine Kugel ist. Das liegt daran, dass sie so groß ist. Ihre Oberfläche ist nur ganz leicht gekrümmt. Außerdem ist sie nicht glatt, es gibt Berge und Schluchten, dadurch kann man die Krümmung nicht sehen.

Unsere Vorfahren haben lange gedacht, dass die **Erde** eine Scheibe ist, über der sich mehrere Glasschalen wölben, an denen Sonne, Mond und **Sterne** aufgehängt sind.

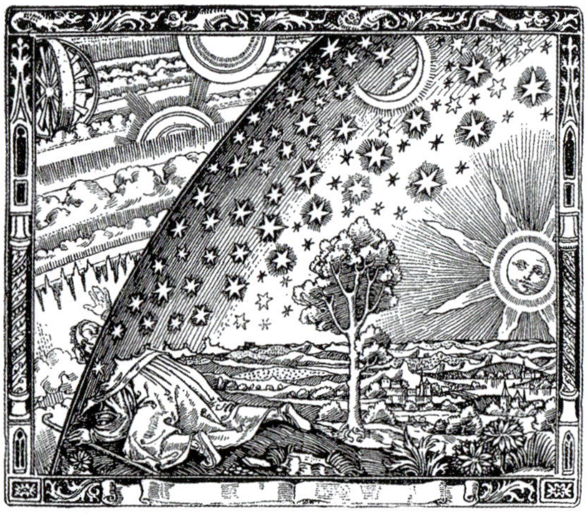

Doch vor etwa 2.500 Jahren bekamen die Menschen Zweifel, ob das wirklich stimmte. Die Kapitäne hatten beobachtet, dass man von einem wegfahrenden Schiff die Segel noch sieht, während der untere Teil schon hinter dem Horizont verschwunden ist.

1 **So sieht das Schiff aus der Nähe aus.**

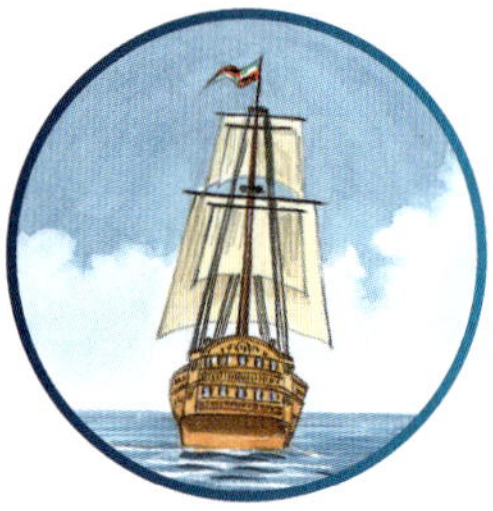

2 **Das Schiff hat sich so weit entfernt, dass der untere Teil vom Horizont verdeckt wird.**

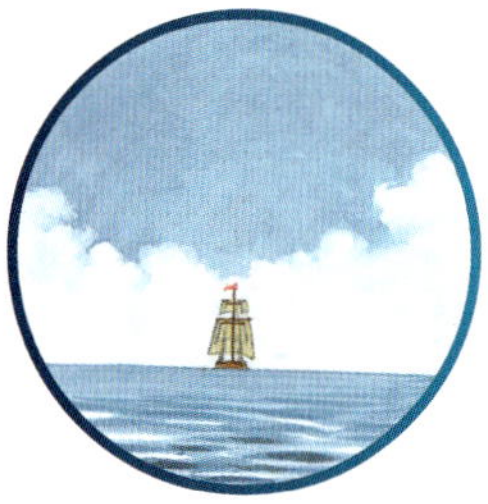

3 **Bald darauf ist das Schiff fast ganz hinter dem Horizont verschwunden.**

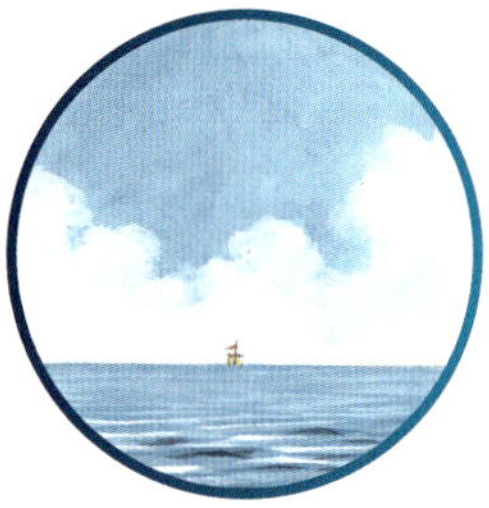

4

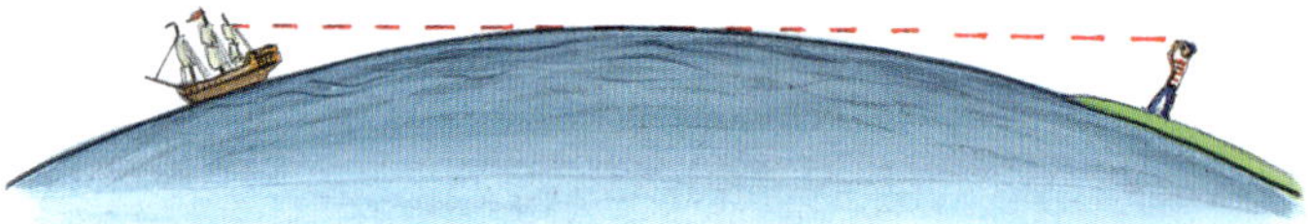

Das Schiff verschwindet hinter der Krümmung der Erdoberfläche.

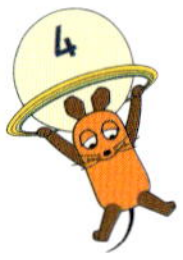

Außerdem tauchten, je weiter man nach Süden fuhr, ganz neue **Sterne** und **Sternbilder** auf. Bei einer scheibenförmigen Erde hätten die Sternbilder immer gleich bleiben müssen.

Der griechische Gelehrte Aristoteles veröffentlichte diese und andere Beweise für eine kugelförmige Erde.

Viel schwieriger war es zu beweisen, dass die Erde sich um die Sonne dreht. Denn für die meisten Leute war damals ganz klar, dass unsere Welt im Mittelpunkt des **Universums** steht.
Nikolaus Kopernikus behauptete im Jahr 1514 zum ersten Mal, dass es nicht so ist. Sehr lange wollten die Menschen das nicht glauben.

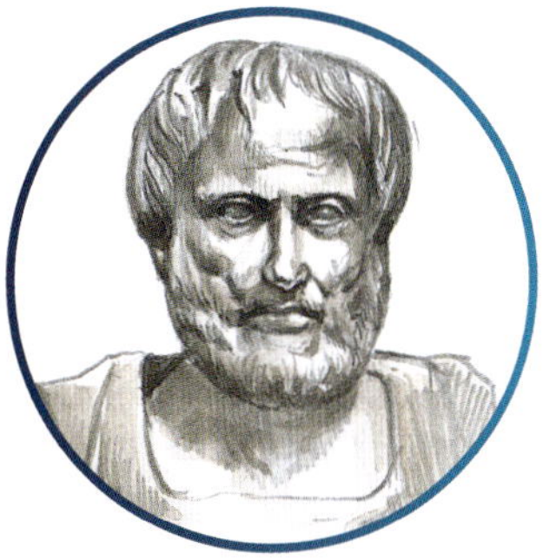

Das ist Aristoteles. Er lebte von 384 bis 322 vor Christus.

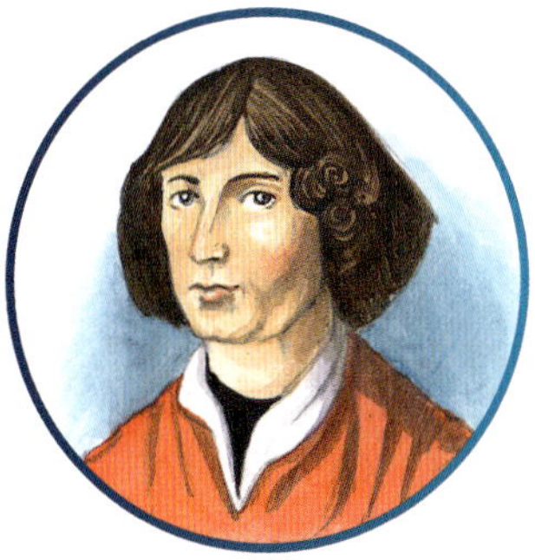

Nikolaus Kopernikus lebte von 1473 bis 1543.

Im Mittelalter wusste jeder gebildete Mensch, dass die Erde eine Kugel ist. Aber erst vor etwa 500 Jahren, gelang es dem portugiesischen Seefahrer Magellan, einmal rund um die Welt zu segeln. Damit überzeugte er auch die letzten Zweifler.

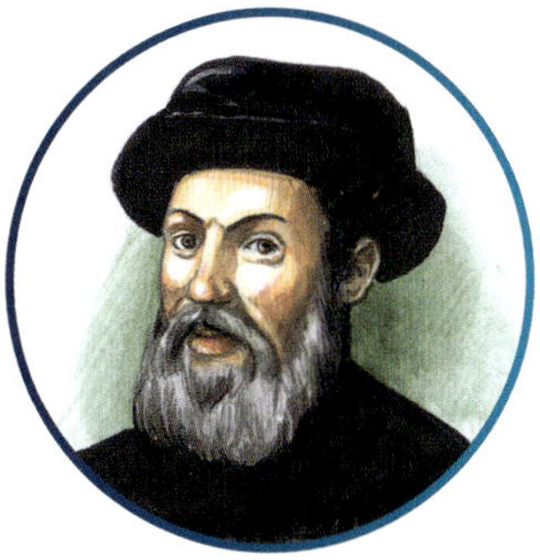

Ferdinand Magellan wurde 1480 geboren und 1521 auf seiner Reise um die Welt bei einem Kampf getötet.

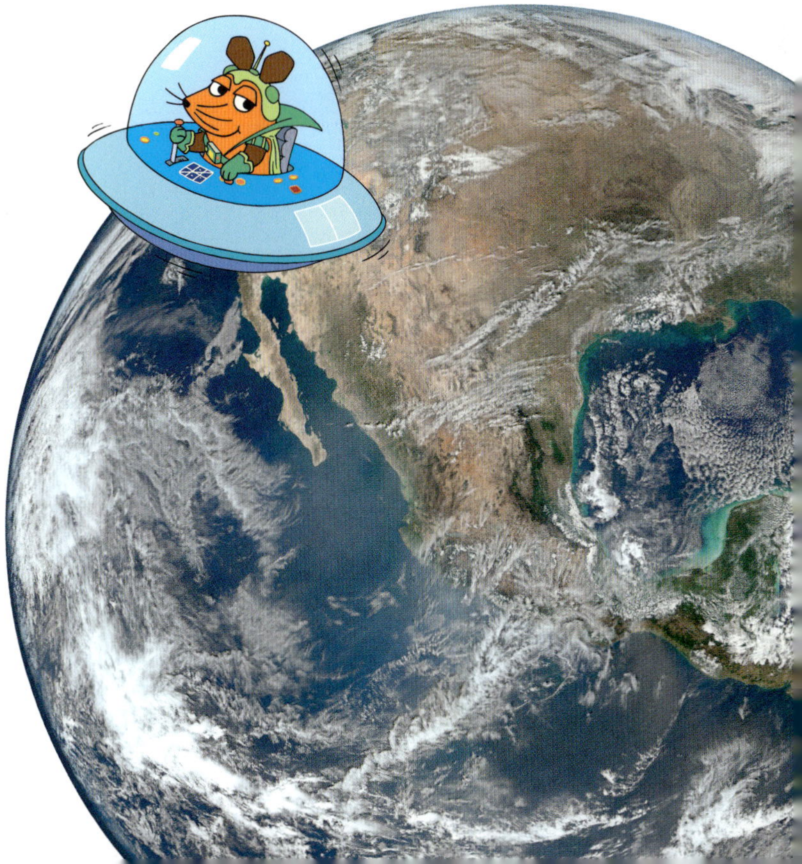

Warum merkt man nicht, dass sich die Erde so schnell dreht?

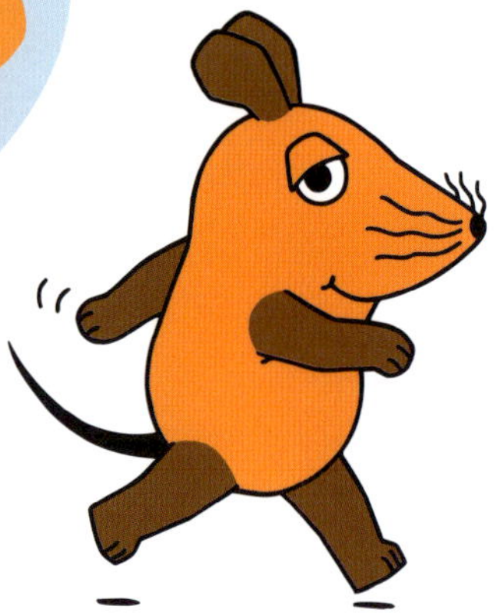

Die Erde dreht sich in 24 Stunden einmal um ihre Achse. Ein Mensch am Äquator legt in dieser Zeit einen viel weiteren Weg zurück als ein Mensch, der näher am Nordpol steht. Darum ist die Geschwindigkeit je nach Ort verschieden. In Hamburg dreht sich die Erde mit 995 Stundenkilometern um sich selbst, in München mit 1.117, am Äquator sogar mit 1.674 Stundenkilometern. Fast doppelt so schnell, wie ein großes Düsenflugzeug fliegt!

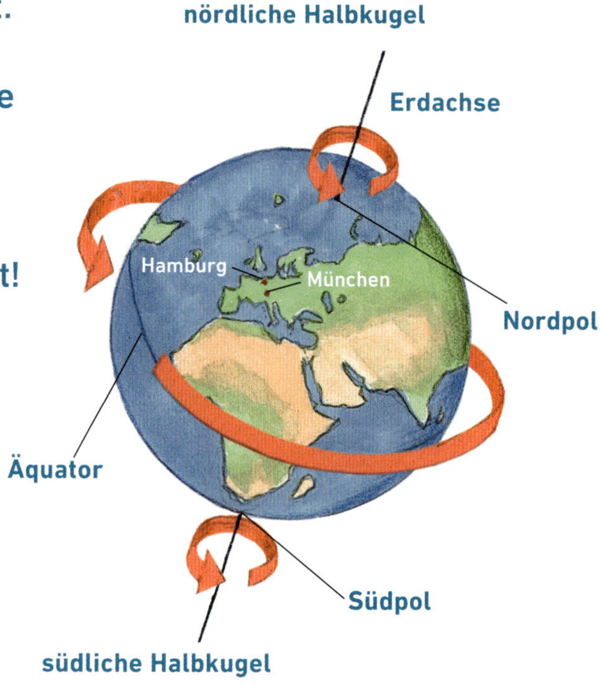

Es hängt aber immer von der Umgebung ab, ob man seine eigene Geschwindigkeit bemerkt. Stell dir vor, du sitzt im Zug und schaust aus dem Fenster. Draußen siehst du Häuser, Wiesen und Felder vorbeisausen. Wenn du das Fenster aufmachst, spürst du den Fahrtwind. Durch den Vergleich mit der Welt draußen kannst du feststellen, dass du dich schnell bewegst.

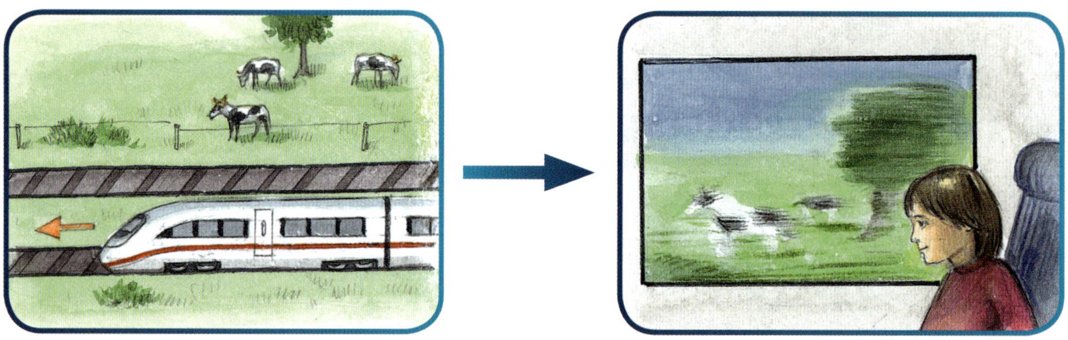

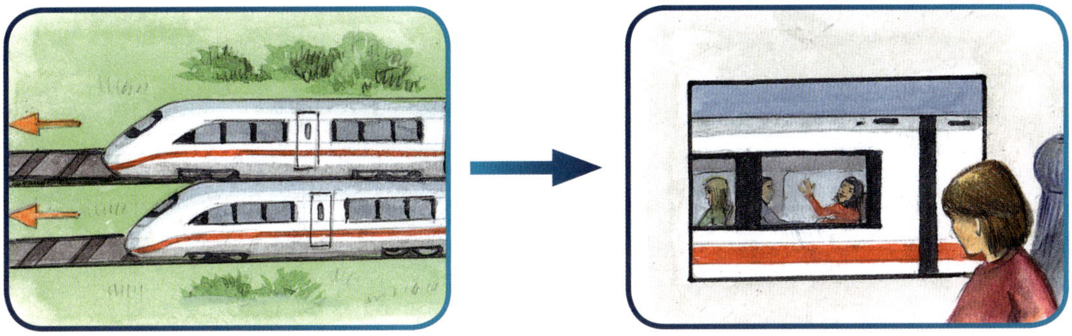

Nun wird dein Zug von einem anderen eingeholt. Eine Zeit lang fahren beide Züge genau nebeneinander Du siehst in dem anderen Zug ein Mädchen am Fenster sitzen. Eine Minute lang gibt es draußen vor deinem Fenster keine Bewegung. Du merkst die Geschwindigkeit nicht mehr. Du könntest glauben, dass dein Zug steht, und der andere Zug auch. Ähnlich ist es bei der **Erde**. Nicht nur wir bewegen uns, sondern auch alles andere auf der Erdoberfläche bewegt sich, sogar die Lufthülle. Also gibt es keinen Fahrtwind! Dass unsere Lufthülle nicht einfach wegfliegt, während die Erde sich dreht, hängt mit der **Schwerkraft** (auch Anziehungskraft genannt) zusammen. Jede große Masse zieht andere Dinge in ihrer Umgebung an, das ist ein Naturgesetz. Deshalb hält die Erde die Luft um sich herum fest.

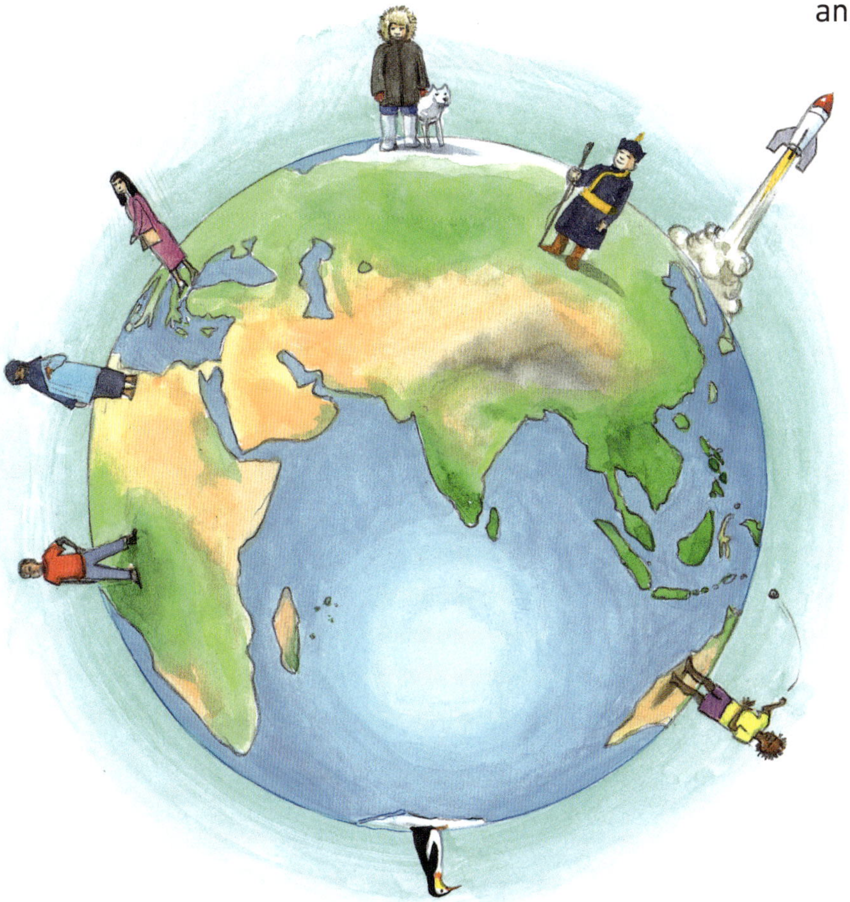

Die Schwerkraft ist auch der Grund, warum Menschen, die auf der südlichen Hälfte der Erde wohnen, nicht herunterfallen.

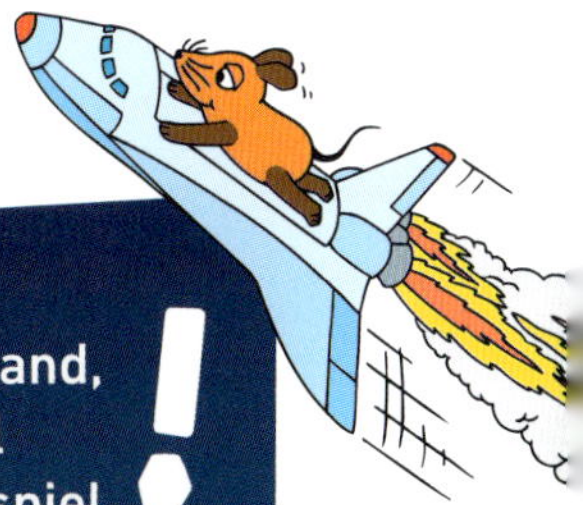

Nur ein Gegenstand, der sehr schnell fliegt – zum Beispiel eine Rakete – kann die Schwerkraft der Erde überwinden.

Warum fällt uns der Mond nicht auf den Kopf?

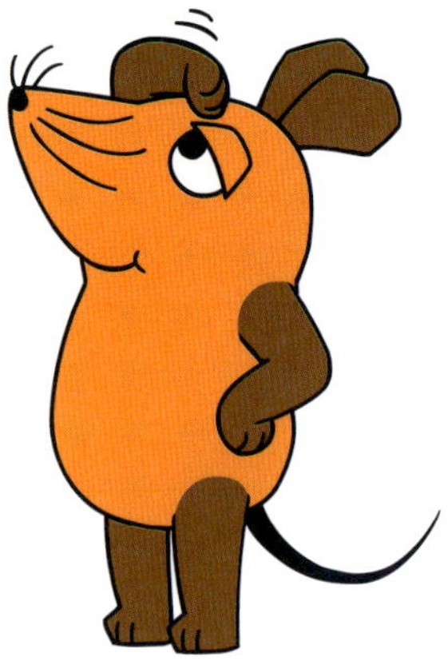

Manchmal steht der Mond so groß, rund und gelb am Himmel, dass es aussieht, als würde er jeden Moment herunterfallen. Doch das wird nicht passieren.

Zwar wird der Mond durch die **Schwerkraft** zur Erde hingezogen, aber eine zweite Kraft drängt ihn wieder von der Erde weg. Diese Kraft kannst du in einem kleinen Versuch kennenlernen. Binde einen Gegenstand, zum Beispiel einen Radiergummi, an eine Schnur und schleudere ihn daran im Kreis herum. Dieser Schwung drängt den Radiergummi nach außen – er würde wegfliegen, wenn du loslassen würdest. Das, was auf ihn einwirkt, nennt man **Fliehkraft**. Der Mond dreht sich ganz schnell um die Erde und ist derselben Kraft ausgesetzt wie der Radiergummi.

Die Schwerkraft der Erde sorgt dafür, dass er nicht davonfliegt (so wie die Schnur den Radiergummi festhält). Da sich beide Kräfte – Fliehkraft und Schwerkraft – die Waage halten, bleibt der Mond auf seiner **Umlaufbahn**. Herunterfallen würde er nur, wenn ihn jemand plötzlich abbremsen würde.

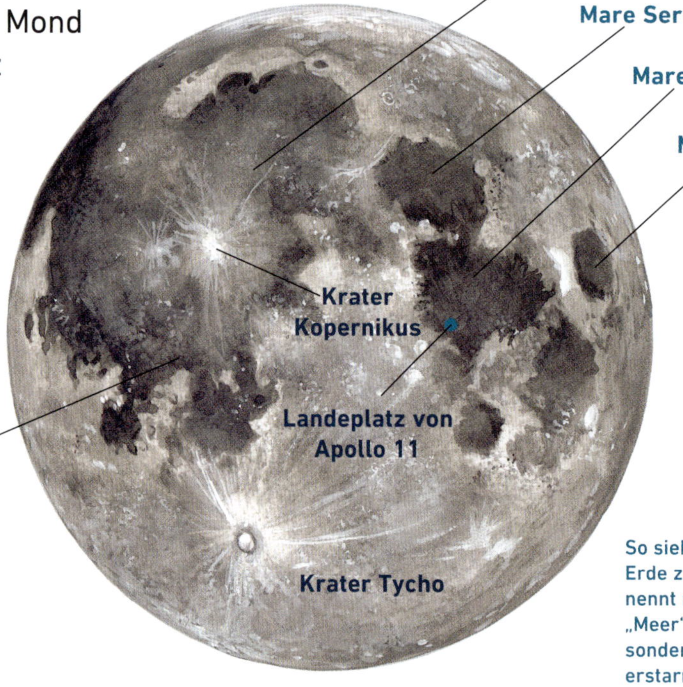

So sieht die Seite des Mondes aus, die der Erde zugewandt ist. Die dunklen Gebiete nennt man „Mare“, das heißt auf Lateinisch „Meer“. Sie bestehen nicht aus Wasser, sondern aus geschmolzenem und wieder erstarrtem Vulkangestein.

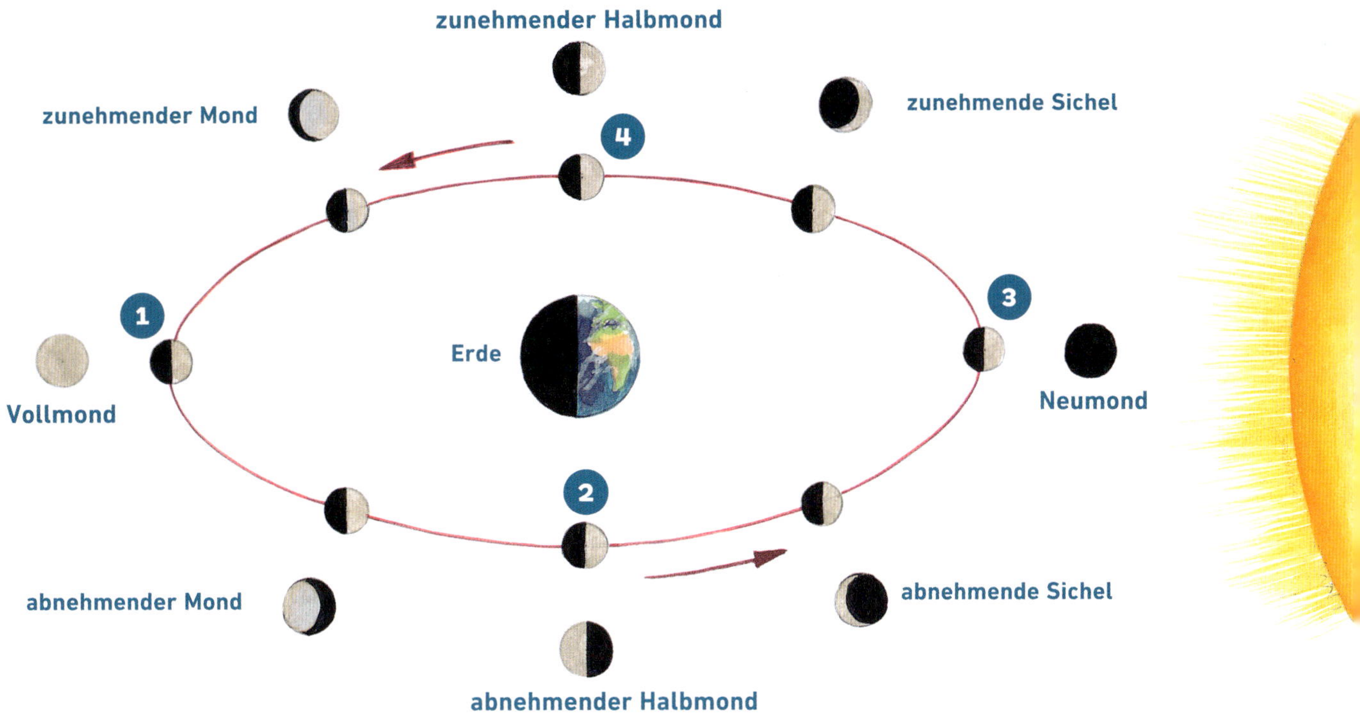

Die kreisförmige Linie ist die Bahn, auf der sich der Mond um die Erde bewegt. An den kleinen Monden auf dem Kreis kannst du sehen, wie der Mond auf seinem Weg von der Sonne angestrahlt wird. Die Zeichnungen daneben zeigen, wie der Mond – von der Erde aus betrachtet – aussieht.

1 Manchmal sehen wir die beleuchtete Seite des Mondes ganz, dann ist Vollmond.

2 Ein paar Tage später sehen wir sie von der Seite und am Himmel ist nur ein halber Mond zu sehen. Es ist der „abnehmende Halbmond".

3 Bei Neumond ist die helle Seite des Mondes von der Erde abgewandt, sodass wir den Mond gar nicht sehen können.

4 Bald ist wieder Halbmond. Diesmal wird der Mond von Tag zu Tag etwas voller und heißt deshalb „zunehmender Halbmond".

Der Mond sieht jede Nacht anders aus. Das liegt daran, dass er nicht selbst leuchtet. Er wirft nur das Sonnenlicht zurück. Hell ist er immer auf der Seite, die gerade von der Sonne beschienen wird, die andere Seite liegt im Schatten.

Als die **Astronauten** vom Mond aus auf die Erde geschaut haben, sahen sie das alles übrigens genau umgekehrt: Vollerde, Halberde und so weiter.

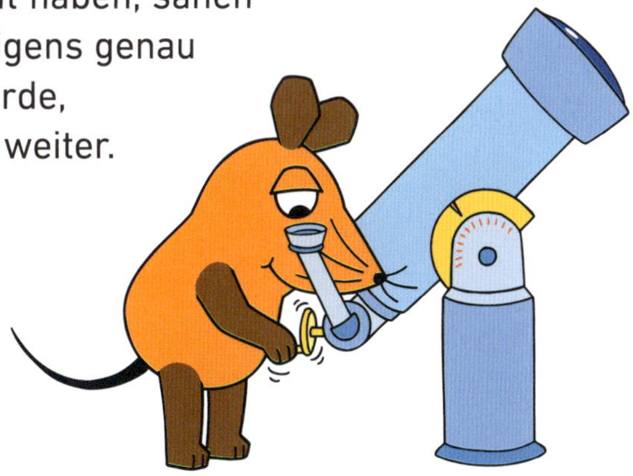

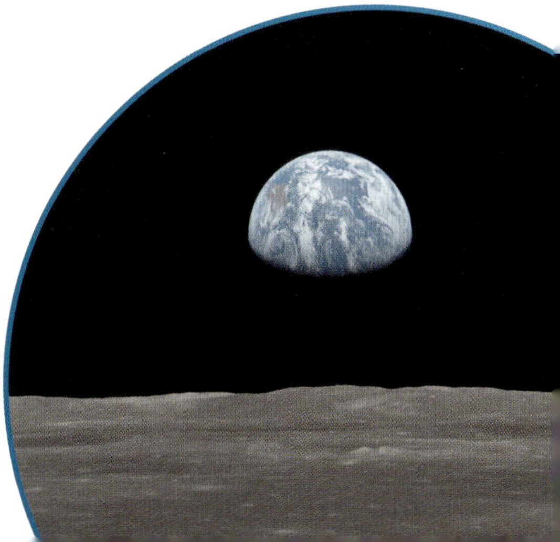

Warum ist man im Weltall schwerelos?

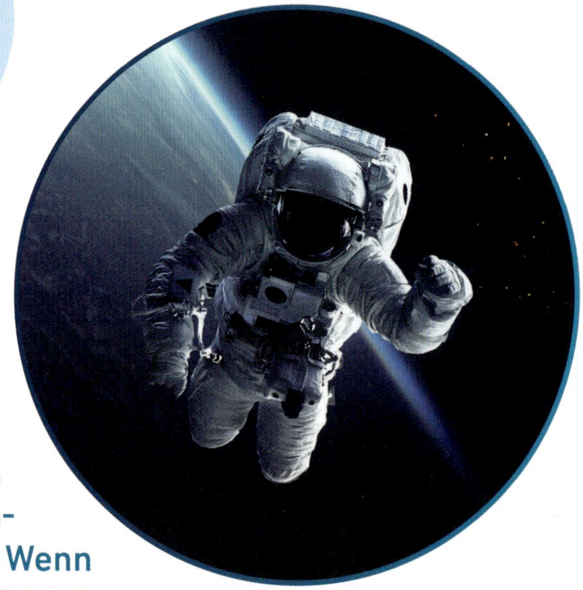

Die Schwerkraft der Erde zieht uns nach unten und hält uns auf dem Boden. Aber im Weltall, zwischen den Sternen und Planeten, ist die Schwerkraft meist sehr schwach, deshalb gibt es kein Oben und Unten. Das heißt: Wenn nichts in der Nähe ist, das Schwerkraft ausübt, ist man schwerelos und schwebt im All.

Anders ist es bei einem **Raumschiff**, das um die Erde kreist. In seiner Flughöhe ist die Schwerkraft fast genauso stark wie am Erdboden. Trotzdem schweben die **Astronauten** in dem Raumschiff.

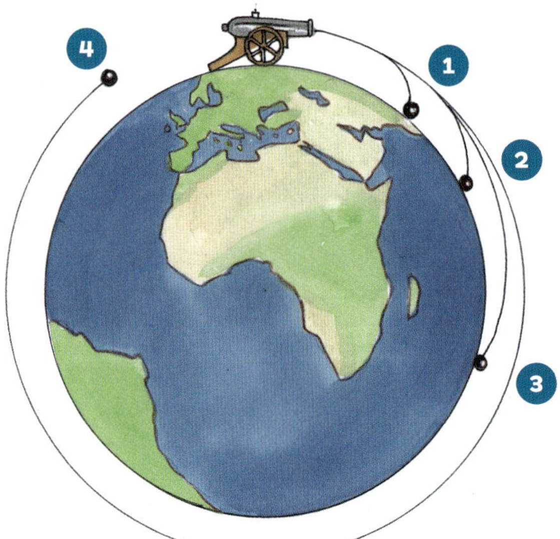

Um zu verstehen, warum das so ist, kannst du dir Folgendes vorstellen: Du baust auf einem sehr, sehr hohen Berg eine Kanone auf. Erst feuerst du deine Kanone mit wenig Schießpulver ab – die Kugel fliegt in einem kurzen Bogen und fällt dann zu Boden 1.
Beim zweiten Schuss nimmst du mehr Schießpulver, dadurch fliegt die Kugel schneller und fällt in einem weiten Bogen auch herunter 2. Ebenso die schneller fliegende dritte Kugel 3.
Die vierte Kugel feuerst du mit so viel Schießpulver ab, dass sie immer weiter und weiter fliegt ... Sie bewegt sich um die Erde herum 4.
Jetzt wirken die gleichen Kräfte, die auch den Mond auf seiner Bahn um die Erde halten. Die **Schwerkraft**, die

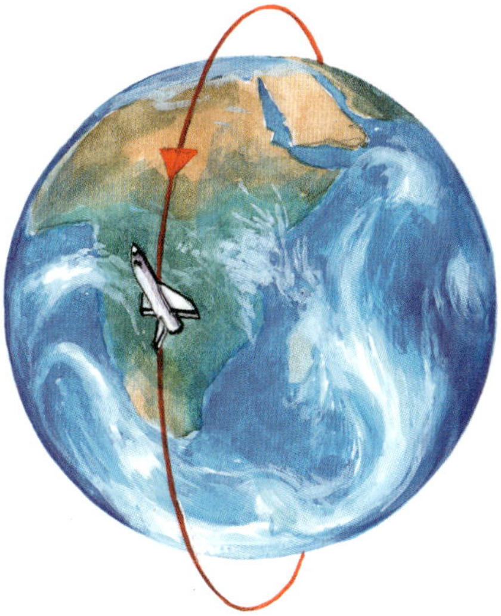

die Kanonenkugel nach unten zieht, und die **Fliehkraft**, die die Kugel nach außen drückt, sind gleich stark und heben sich dadurch gegenseitig auf. In einer solchen Umlaufbahn bewegt sich ein Raumschiff. Es kann monatelang um die Erde „herumfallen“. Und da alles, was es enthält, genauso schnell fällt wie das Raumschiff selbst, sind die **Astronauten** an Bord schwerelos.

Auch auf der Erde kannst du ein paar Sekunden lang schwerelos sein. Zum Beispiel auf dem Jahrmarkt. Dort gibt es Geräte, die wie hohe Türme aussehen. Du wirst auf einem Sitz festgeschnallt und den Turm hochgefahren. Dann fällst du ganz plötzlich in die Tiefe und bist ein, zwei Sekunden lang schwerelos!

Setzte man dich auf eine Waage, würde sie in diesem Moment null anzeigen. Sie fällt nämlich genauso schnell wie du, dein Gewicht kann nicht auf sie drücken. Deshalb nennt man Schwerelosigkeit auch **Freier Fall**.

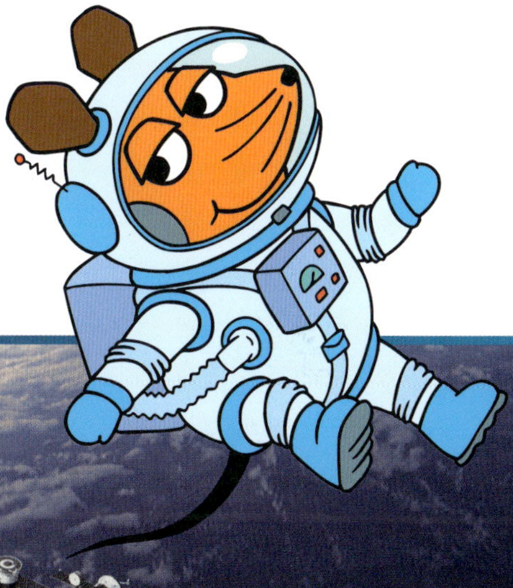

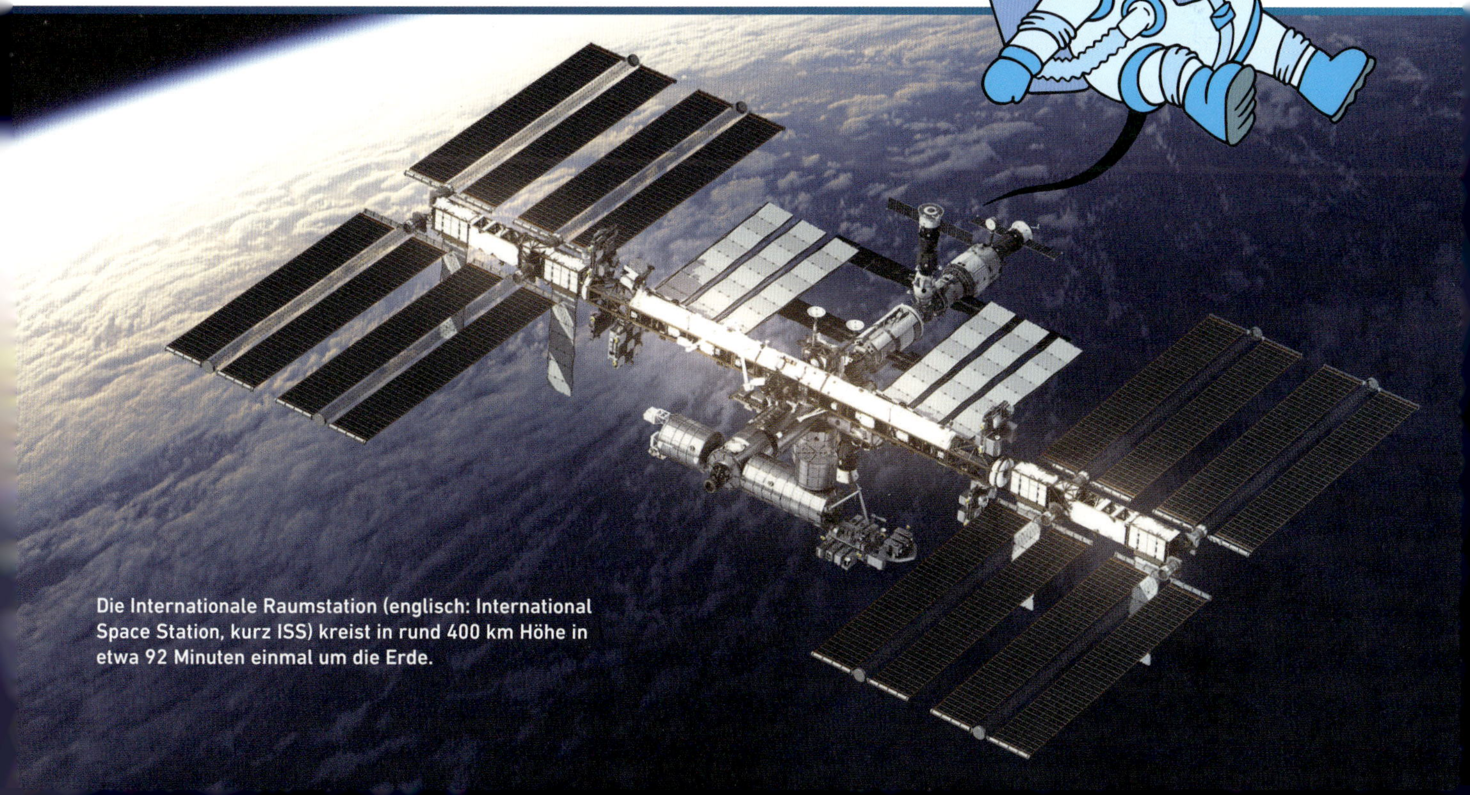

Die Internationale Raumstation (englisch: International Space Station, kurz ISS) kreist in rund 400 km Höhe in etwa 92 Minuten einmal um die Erde.

Warum ist die Sonne gelb?

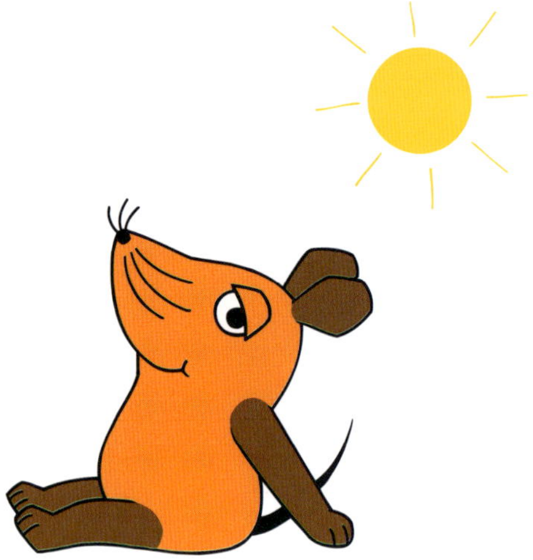

Sterne wie unsere Sonne sind gigantische Kugeln aus glühenden Gasen. Ihre Farbe hängt von der Temperatur ab, die sie haben.

Der Stern, den wir **Sonne** nennen, hat eine mittlere Temperatur – und ist deshalb gelb. Wäre unsere Sonne kühler, würde sie rot leuchten. Wäre sie heißer, hätte sie eine weiße oder bläulich bis weiße Farbe.

Aus dem Kern steigt die Hitze der Sonne langsam durch verschiedene Schichten an die Oberfläche. In ihrer äußeren Hülle brodelt es heftig. Dort entstehen immer wieder riesige **Gasfackeln**.

Die Hitze der Sonne entsteht in ihrem Kern. Im Inneren sind Hitze und Druck so hoch, dass die Teilchen (Atome) verschmelzen – dadurch bekommt die Sonne ihre enorme Energie. Im Kern der Sonne ist es 15.500.000 Grad heiß, auf der Oberfläche immerhin noch 5.500 Grad. Zum Vergleich: Ein gewöhnlicher Backofen kommt auf gerade mal 250 Grad, und Eisen schmilzt bei 1535 Grad.

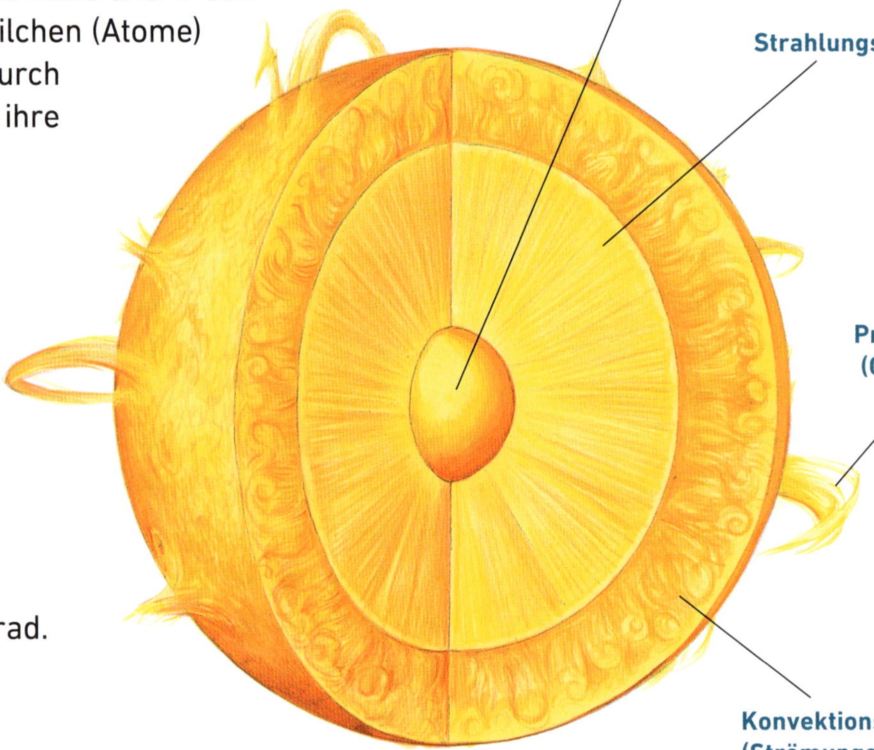

So sieht die Sonne im Querschnitt aus.

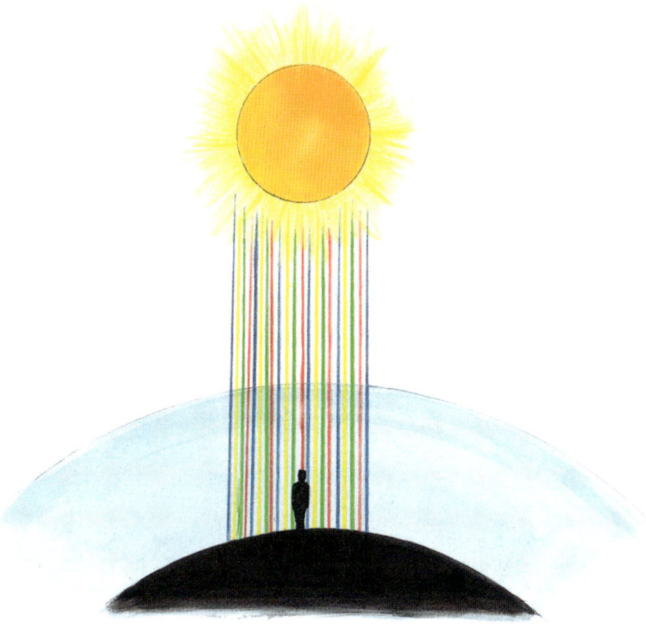

Wenn die Sonne mittags am Himmel steht, muss das Licht nur einen kurzen Weg durch die Lufthülle der Erde zurücklegen. Die Sonne sieht dann gelb aus.

Die Sonne sendet auch unsichtbares ultraviolettes Licht (UV-Licht) aus. Um sich vor diesen schädlichen Strahlen zu schützen, bildet unsere Haut einen dunklen Farbstoff, der das UV-Licht schluckt. Das schafft er nicht lange. Deshalb musst du dich eincremen, damit du keinen Sonnenbrand bekommst. !

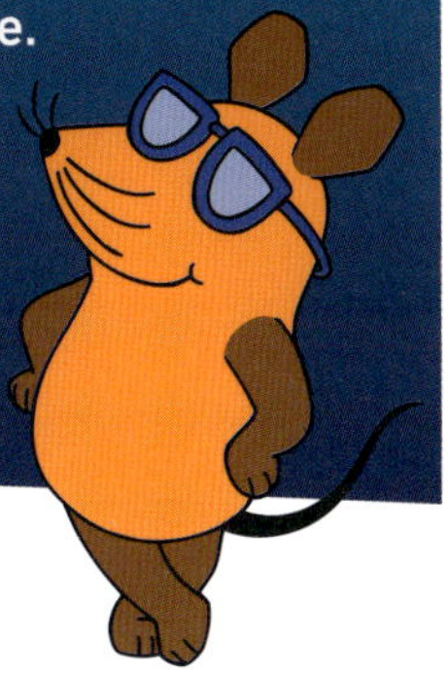

Die Sonne sieht nicht immer gelb aus. Morgens und abends, wenn sie tief über dem Horizont steht, scheint sie rötlich. Das liegt daran, dass, wenn die Sonne tief steht, ihr Licht einen langen Weg durch die Lufthülle der Erde zurücklegen muss. Dabei wird der blaue Teil ihres Lichts von Luftteilchen gestreut. Nur die roten und gelben Teile bleiben übrig, und wir sehen einen tollen **Sonnenuntergang**.

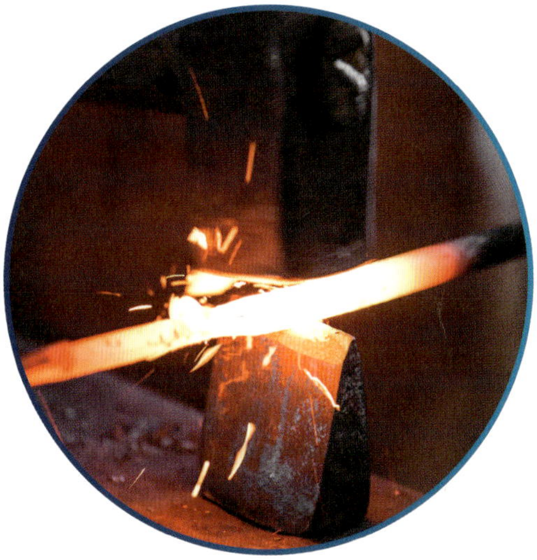

Auch ein Stück Eisen verändert seine Farbe, wenn es erhitzt wird. Während es immer heißer wird, glüht es erst rot, dann orange, dann gelb und schließlich weiß.

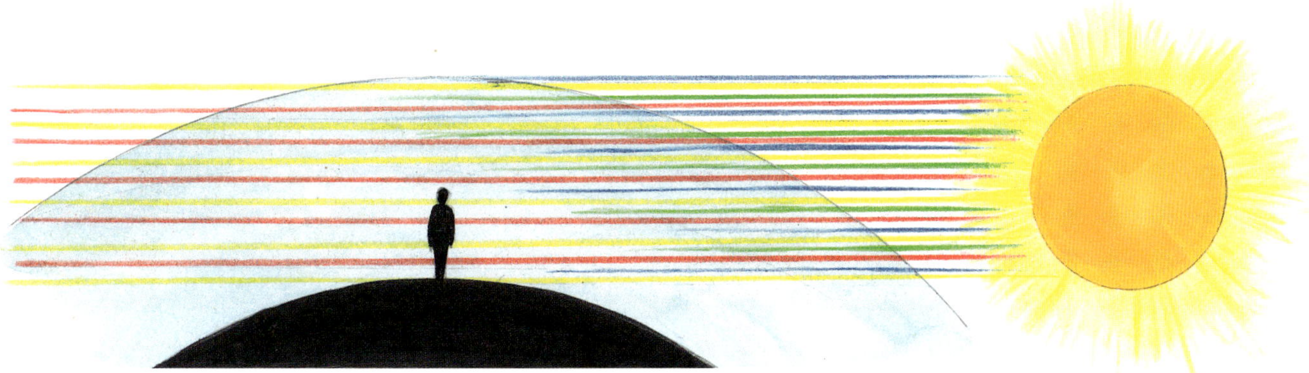

Wenn die Sonne tief steht, siehst du sie durch eine dicke Luftschicht hindurch. Dadurch sieht sie rot aus.

Wie entsteht eine Sonnenfinsternis?

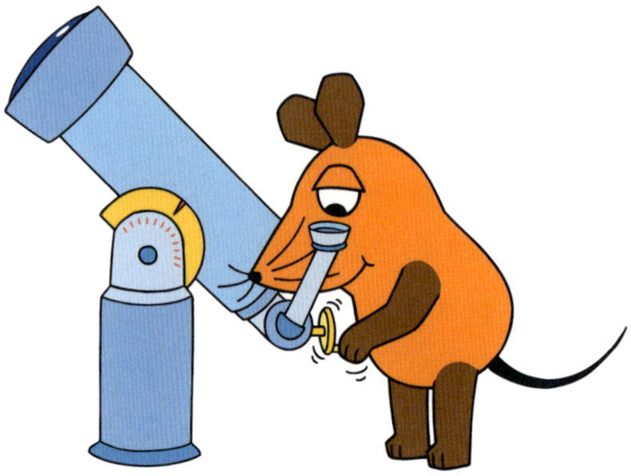

Eine Sonnenfinsternis entsteht, wenn der Mond auf seiner Bahn direkt vor der Sonne vorbeizieht und sie dabei verdeckt. Dort, wo sein Schatten auf die Erde fällt, sieht man die Sonnenfinsternis.

Wenn die Sonnenscheibe ganz verschwindet, sodass es mitten am Tag für ein paar Minuten dunkel wird, spricht man von einer „totalen **Sonnenfinsternis**“. Sonnenfinsternisse sind gar nicht so selten. Fast jedes Jahr gibt es eine oder mehrere, nur sieht man sie nicht von jeder Gegend der Erde aus. Die nächste totale Sonnenfinsternis kannst du in Deutschland am 3. September 2081 beobachten. Um eine Finsternis zu beobachten, brauchst du eine spezielle Sonnenfinsternis-Brille. Ohne sie solltest du nie direkt in die Sonne schauen, das ist sehr schädlich für deine Augen.

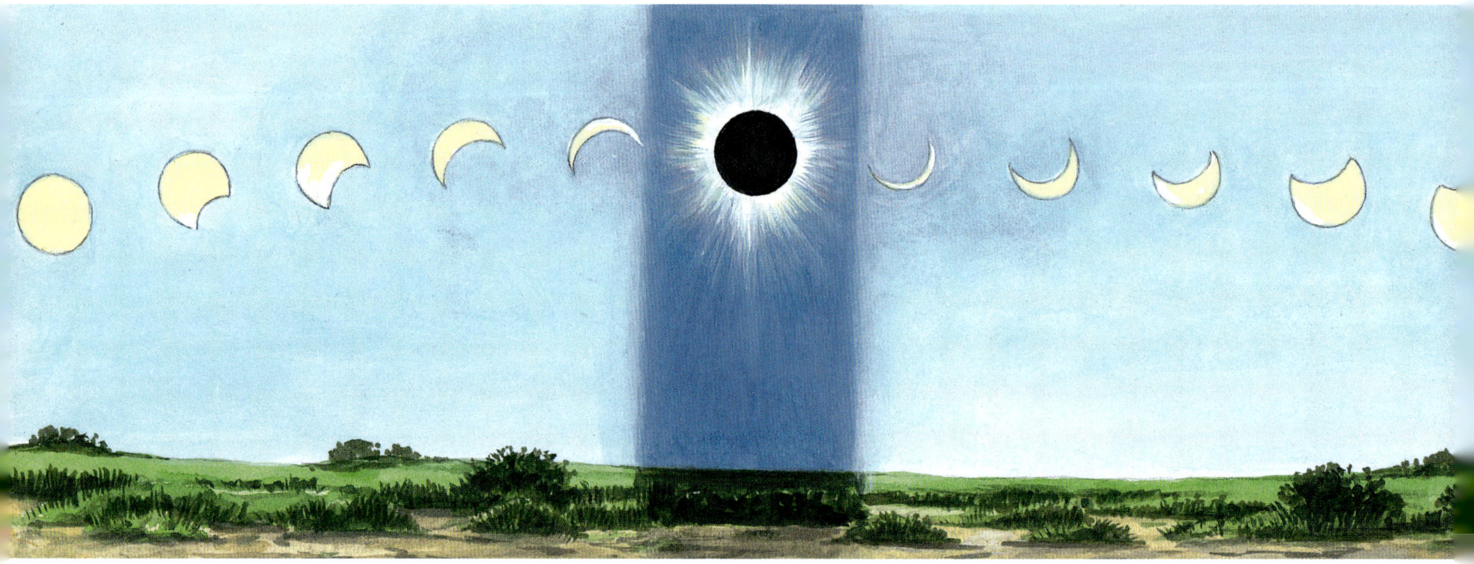

Langsam schiebt sich der Mond vor die Sonne, das nennt man Sonnenfinsternis. Danach entfernt sich der Mond wieder und die Sonnenscheibe wird wieder sichtbar.

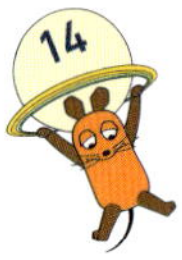

Sonnenfinsternis

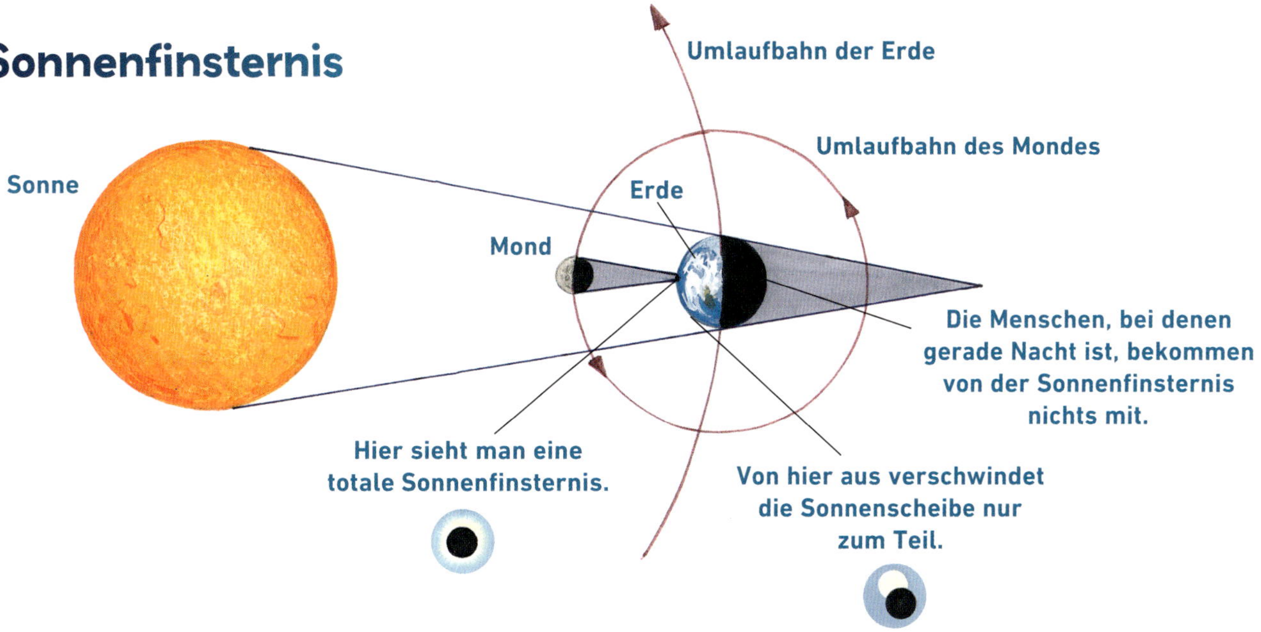
Umlaufbahn der Erde
Umlaufbahn des Mondes
Sonne
Erde
Mond
Die Menschen, bei denen gerade Nacht ist, bekommen von der Sonnenfinsternis nichts mit.
Hier sieht man eine totale Sonnenfinsternis.
Von hier aus verschwindet die Sonnenscheibe nur zum Teil.

Eine **Mondfinsternis** entsteht, wenn der Mond durch den Schatten der Erde wandert. Da die Erde einen großen Schatten wirft, braucht der Mond lange, um ihn zu durchqueren. Deshalb dauert so eine Finsternis bis zu eineinhalb Stunden. Der Mond verschwindet dabei nicht, sondern sieht dunkler oder rötlich aus, weil einige Sonnenstrahlen durch die Lufthülle der Erde dringen und den Mond auch im Schatten noch erreichen. Eine Mondfinsternis kann man von Deutschland aus etwa zweimal im Jahr sehen.

Mondfinsternis

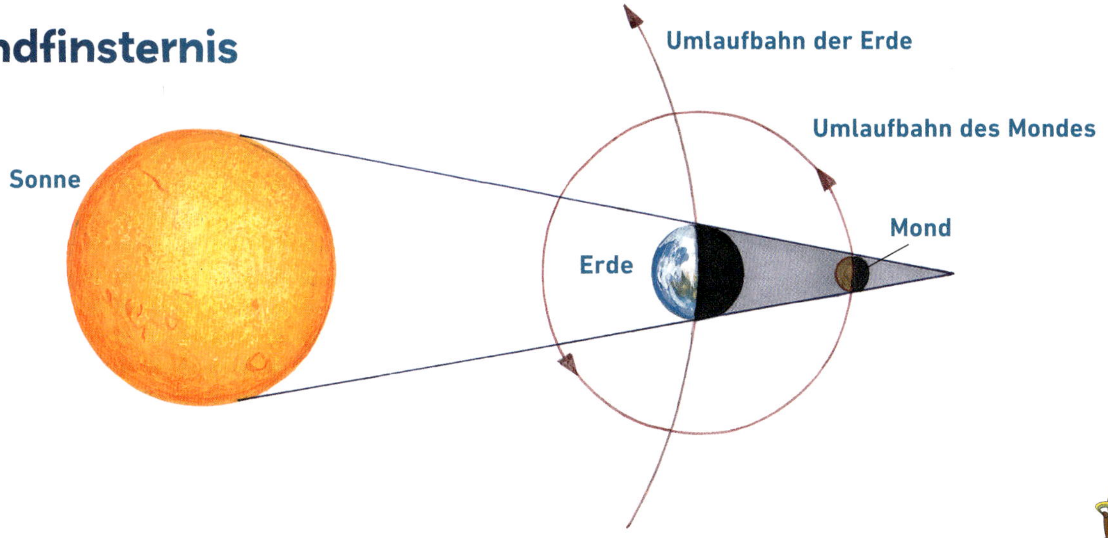
Umlaufbahn der Erde
Umlaufbahn des Mondes
Sonne
Mond
Erde

Wie viele Planeten hat die Sonne?

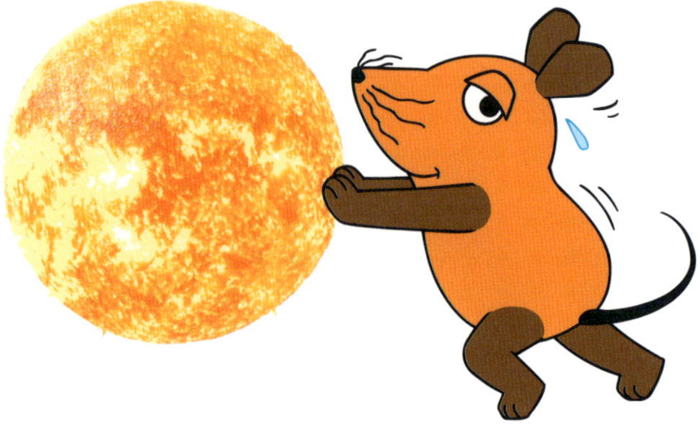

Ein richtiger Planet ist ein großer, runder, nicht leuchtender Himmelskörper, der mit seiner Schwerkraft seine Umgebung beherrscht. Unser Sonnensystem hat acht Planeten.

Gebildet haben sich unsere Sonne und ihre Planeten (das **Sonnensystem**) vor 4,5 Milliarden Jahren aus einer wirbelnden Scheibe von Staub und Gas. So haben die Sonne und ihre Umgebung wahrscheinlich ausgesehen, bevor die Planeten entstanden sind:

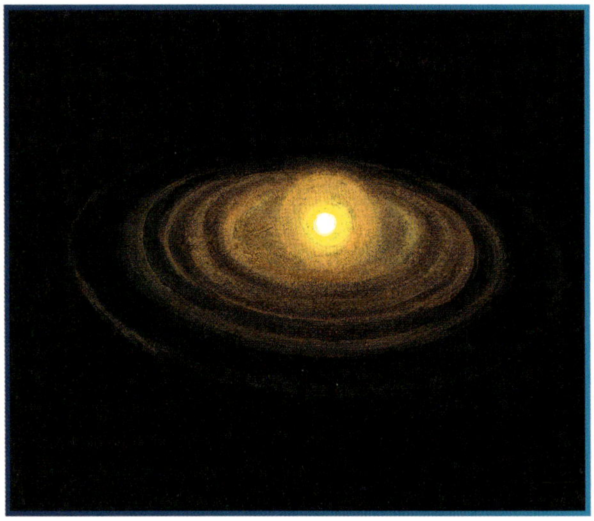

Nach und nach ballten sich Gestein, Staub und Gase zu immer größeren Klumpen zusammen – daraus wurden im Laufe von vielen Millionen Jahren die Planeten. Die vier Planeten, die der Sonne am nächsten sind, bestehen aus Gestein, die anderen aus Gas.

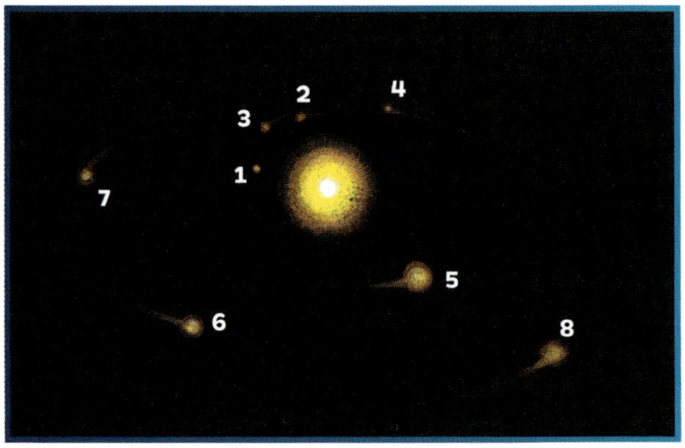

1 Merkur
2 Venus
3 Erde
4 Mars
5 Jupiter
6 Saturn
7 Uranus
8 Neptun

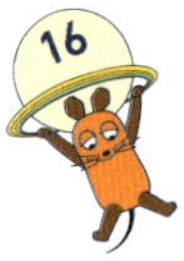

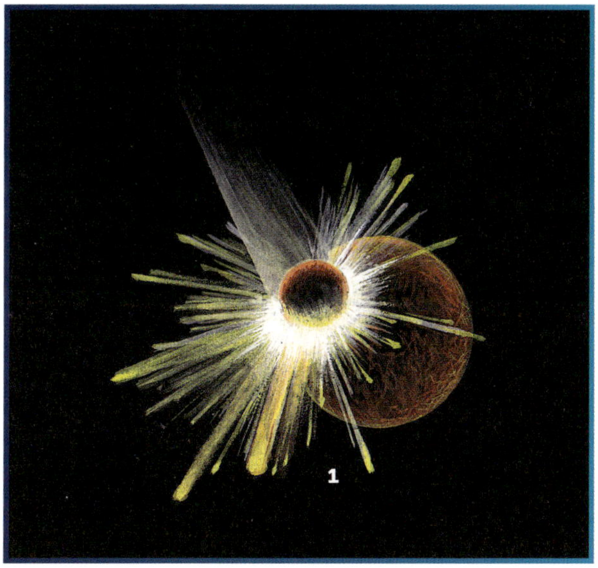

1 Ein Himmelskörper stößt mit hohem Tempo auf unsere Erde.

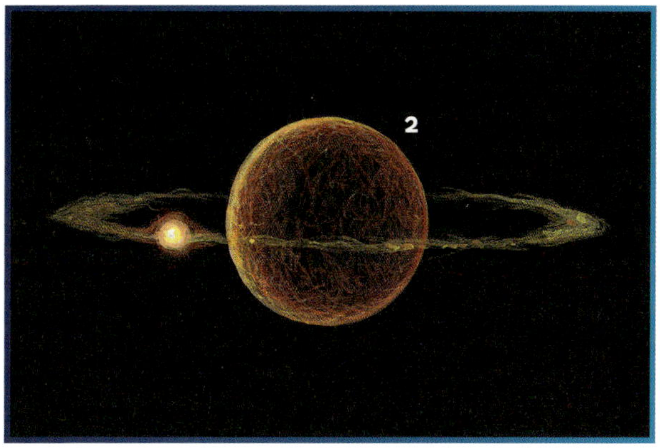

2 Aus den Resten des Himmelskörpers und aus Erdtrümmern ballt sich der Mond zusammen.

Als die Planeten jung waren, flogen sehr viele Gesteinsbrocken durch unser Sonnensystem. Am Merkur und an unserem Mond kann man heute noch sehen, was damals los gewesen sein muss. Überall Krater, die von Treffern stammen.

Die Erde wurde zu dieser Zeit wahrscheinlich von einem Himmelskörper getroffen, der fast so groß gewesen ist wie der Planet Mars. 1 Zum Glück ging die Erde damals nicht kaputt; es wurden nur sehr viele Trümmer hochgeschleudert. Zusammen mit Resten des fremden Himmelskörpers begannen sie die Erde zu umkreisen. Daraus bildete sich unser Mond. 2

Zwischen Mars und Jupiter ist bei der Entstehung der Planeten etwas schiefgegangen. Dort gibt es einen Ring aus Gesteinsbrocken, der **Asteroidengürtel** genannt wird. Ein zweiter Ring, der **Kuiper-Gürtel**, befindet sich hinter dem Planeten Neptun.

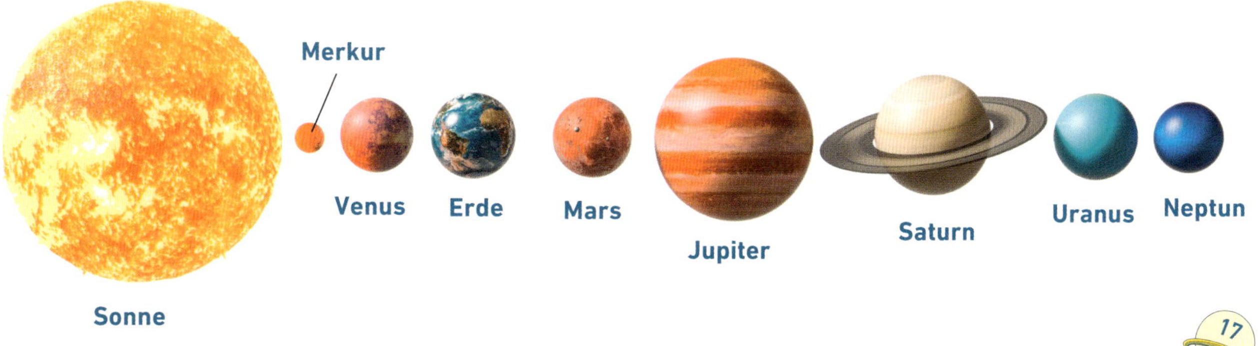

So sieht unser Sonnensystem heute aus:

1 Merkur

Er ist der Sonne am nächsten. Der Merkur hat keine Gashülle, ist von Kratern bedeckt und sieht heute genauso aus wie vor Milliarden von Jahren.

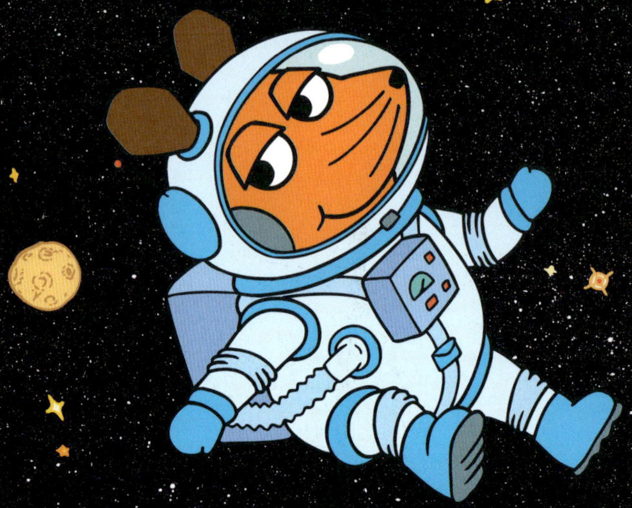

2 Venus

Die Oberfläche der Venus ist unter dichten Wolken, die für uns giftig wären, verborgen. Darunter ist es sehr heiß, denn die Gashülle der Venus heizt sich durch das Sonnenlicht stark auf und gibt die Wärme nicht mehr ab. Unter der Wolkenschicht sind Berge, Vulkane und riesige Ebenen.

3 Erde

Soweit wir wissen, ist die Erde der einzige Planet, auf dem es flüssiges Wasser gibt. Es bedeckt drei Viertel der Erdoberfläche. Außerdem umgibt eine dichte Lufthülle die Erde, die Temperatur ist genau richtig für uns Menschen und alle anderen Lebewesen.

4 Mars

Mars ist ein trockener, kalter Planet aus rötlichem Gestein. Auf seiner Oberfläche toben Staubstürme, die oft monatelang dauern. Er ist nur halb so groß wie die Erde.

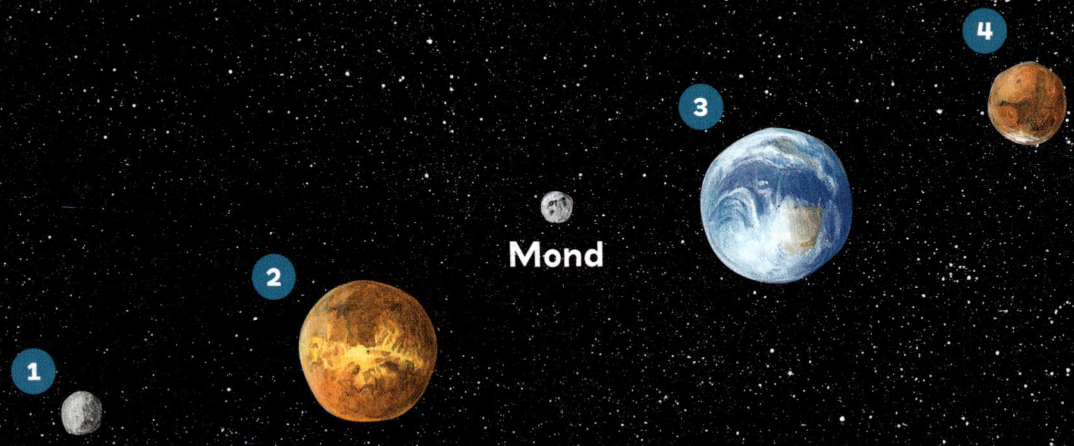

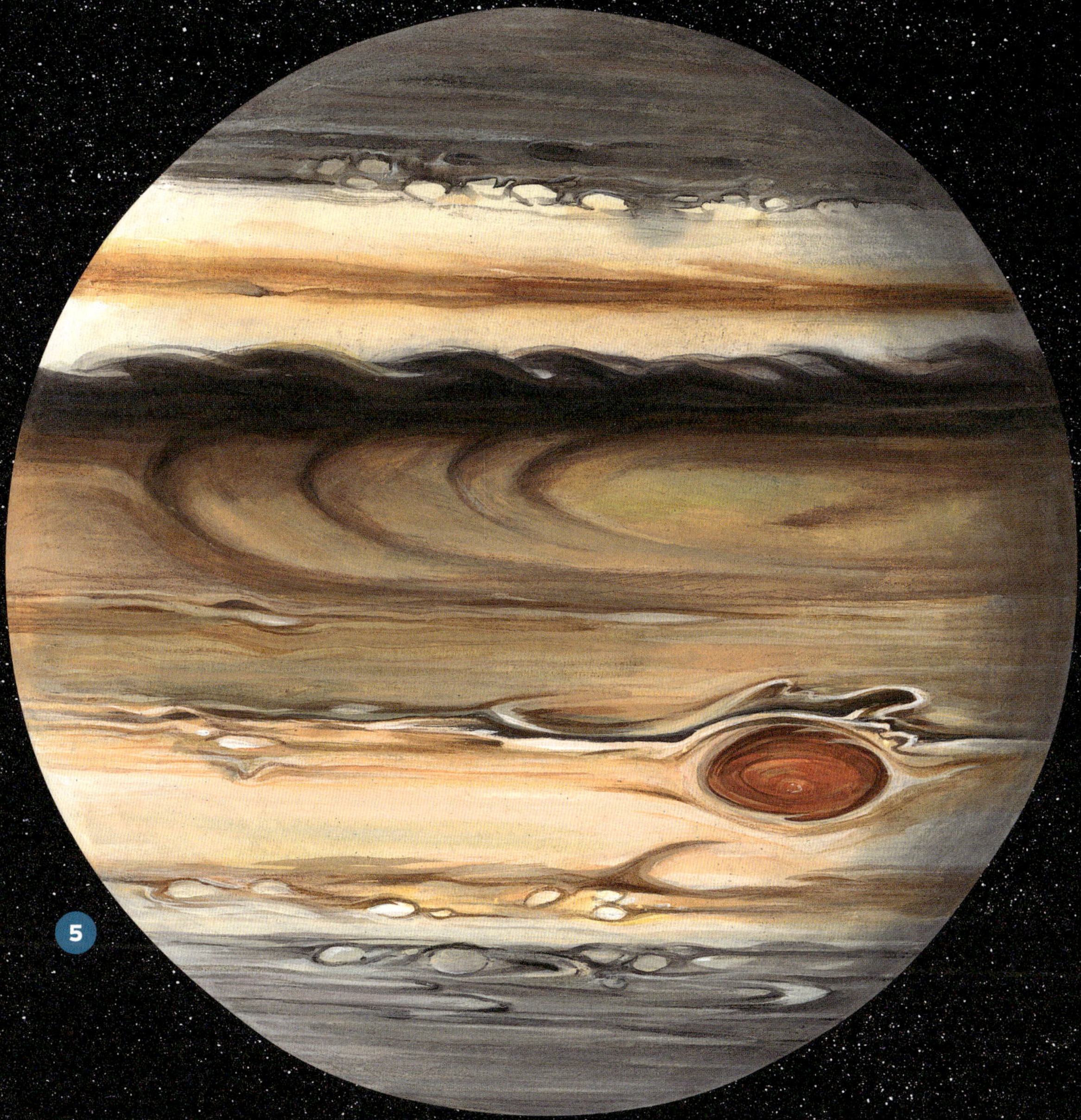

5 Jupiter

Jupiter ist der größte Planet des Sonnensystems und wurde nach dem mächtigsten Gott der alten Römer benannt. Der ganze Planet besteht aus Gas. Jupiter hat sehr viele Monde, 79 kennt man bisher.

7 Uranus

Uranus ist sehr weit von der Sonne entfernt und deshalb sehr kalt. Er besteht aus einem blaugrünen Gasgemisch und hat einen Kern aus schlammigem Eis. Auch Uranus hat Ringe, sie sind aber nur schwach zu sehen.

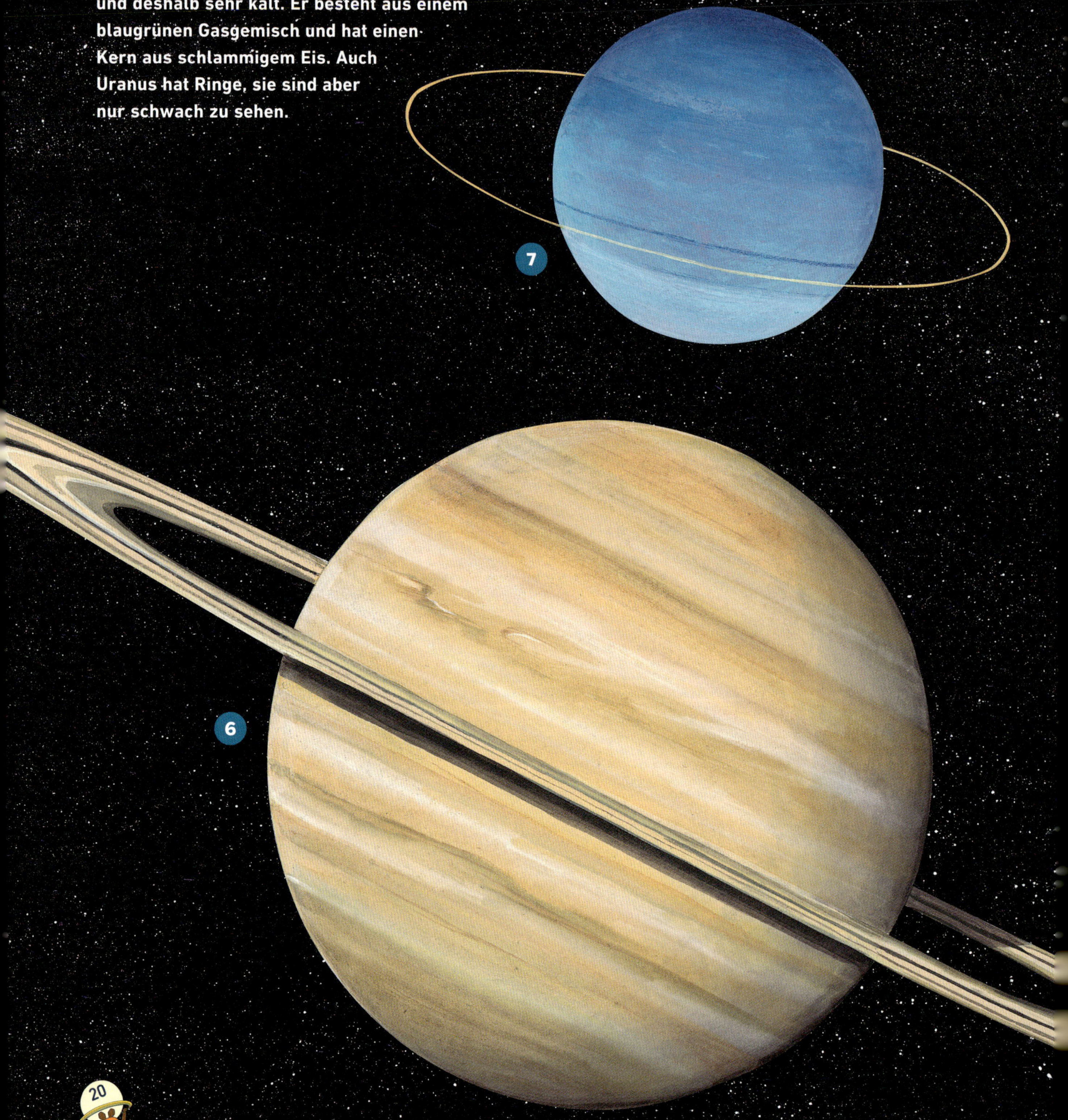

8

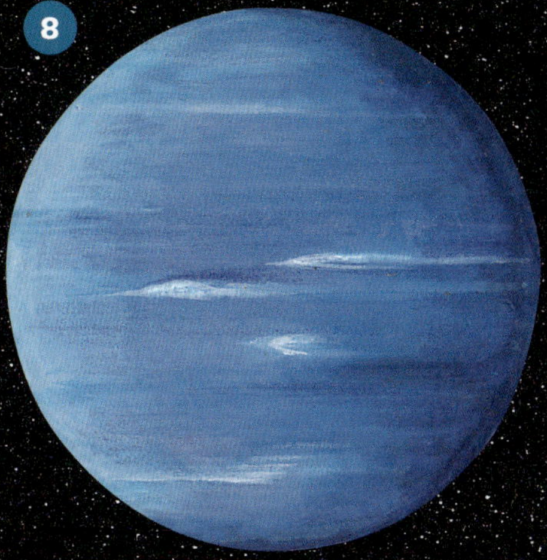

8 Neptun

Er wurde wegen seiner blauen Farbe nach dem römischen Gott des Meeres benannt. Neptun ist ein eisiger Gasplanet, ähnlich wie Uranus. An seiner Oberfläche erkennt man Wolken aus Eiskristallen.

6 Saturn

Der zweitgrößte Planet des Sonnensystems ist bekannt für seine Ringe aus Eis- und Gesteinsbrocken. Auch Saturn besteht aus Gas. Er ist so leicht, dass er auf Wasser schwimmen würde.

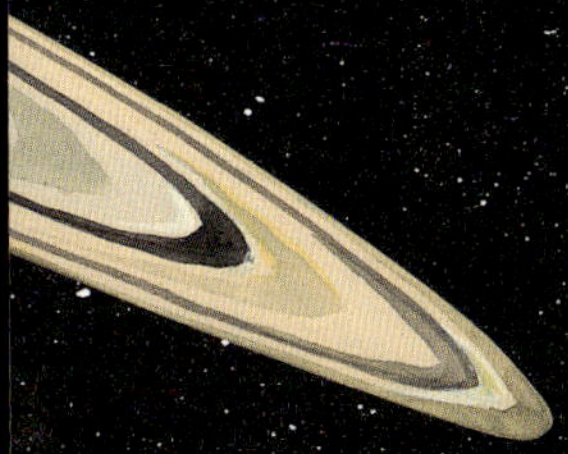

9

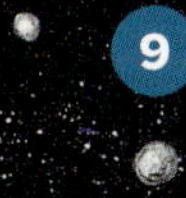

9 Die Zwergplaneten

Pluto ist kleiner als unser Mond und besteht aus Gestein und Eis. Früher galt Pluto als Planet – doch dann entdeckte man in der gleichen Gegend, dem Kuiper-Gürtel, noch Hunderte anderer Gesteinsbrocken. Deshalb gilt er heute nur noch als Zwergplanet. Einen weiteren Zwergplaneten gibt es zwischen Jupiter und Mars, er heißt Ceres.

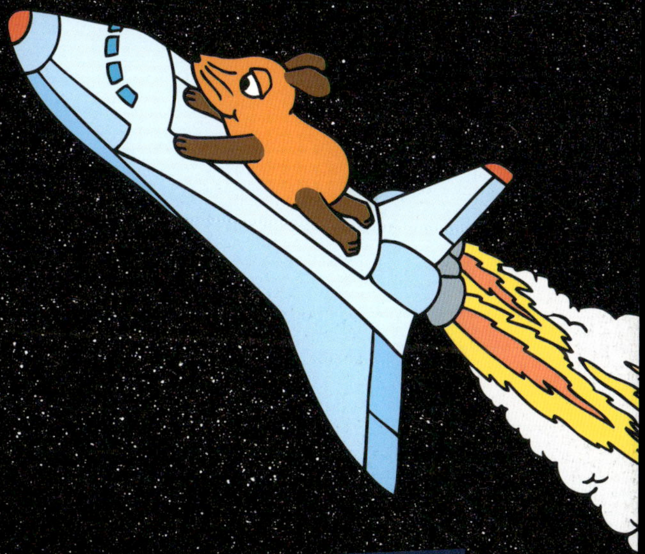

! Die Planeten bewegen sich unterschiedlich schnell und brauchen unterschiedlich lange, um die Sonne einmal zu umrunden: Der Merkur benötigt dafür nur 88 Tage, die Erde ein Jahr und der Jupiter 12 Jahre.

Gibt es Außerirdische?

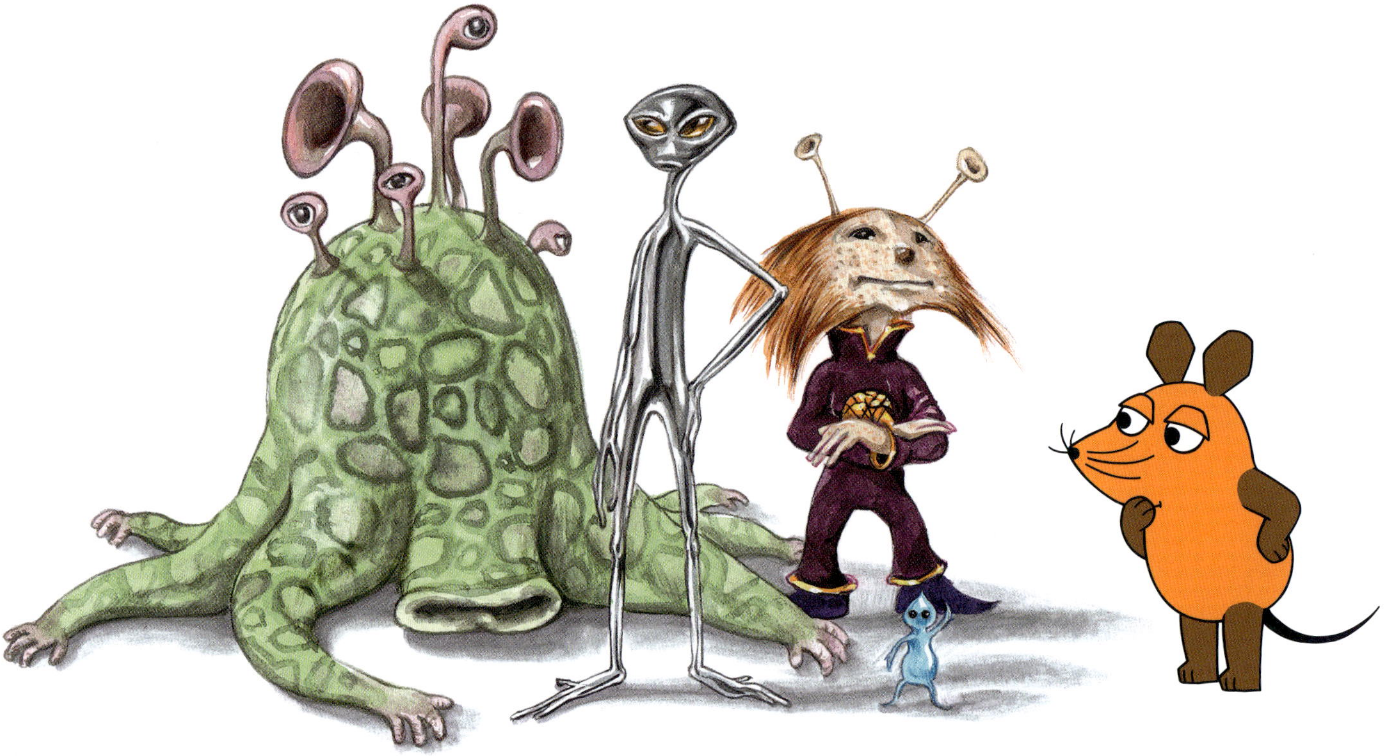

Bisher scheinen noch keine Wesen von anderen Planeten bei uns vorbeigekommen zu sein. Das liegt wahrscheinlich aber nicht daran, dass wir allein im Weltraum sind.

Zwar wohnt auf den anderen **Planeten**, die um unsere Sonne kreisen, niemand. Aber unsere Sonne ist nur einer von sehr vielen Sternen unserer Galaxie. Dies ist eine größere Ansammlung von Sternen, die etwas näher beieinander stehen. In unserer **Galaxie** gibt es ungefähr 100 Milliarden Sterne.

Viele Sterne in unserer Galaxie haben **Planeten**. Obwohl sie sehr klein und schwer zu entdecken sind, hat man bis zum Jahr 2012 schon 716 Planeten gefunden, die andere Sterne umkreisen. Leider ist bisher keiner der Erde ähnlich. Bestimmt gibt es irgendwo im Weltall andere Planeten, auf denen Leben

100 000 000 000 Sterne!

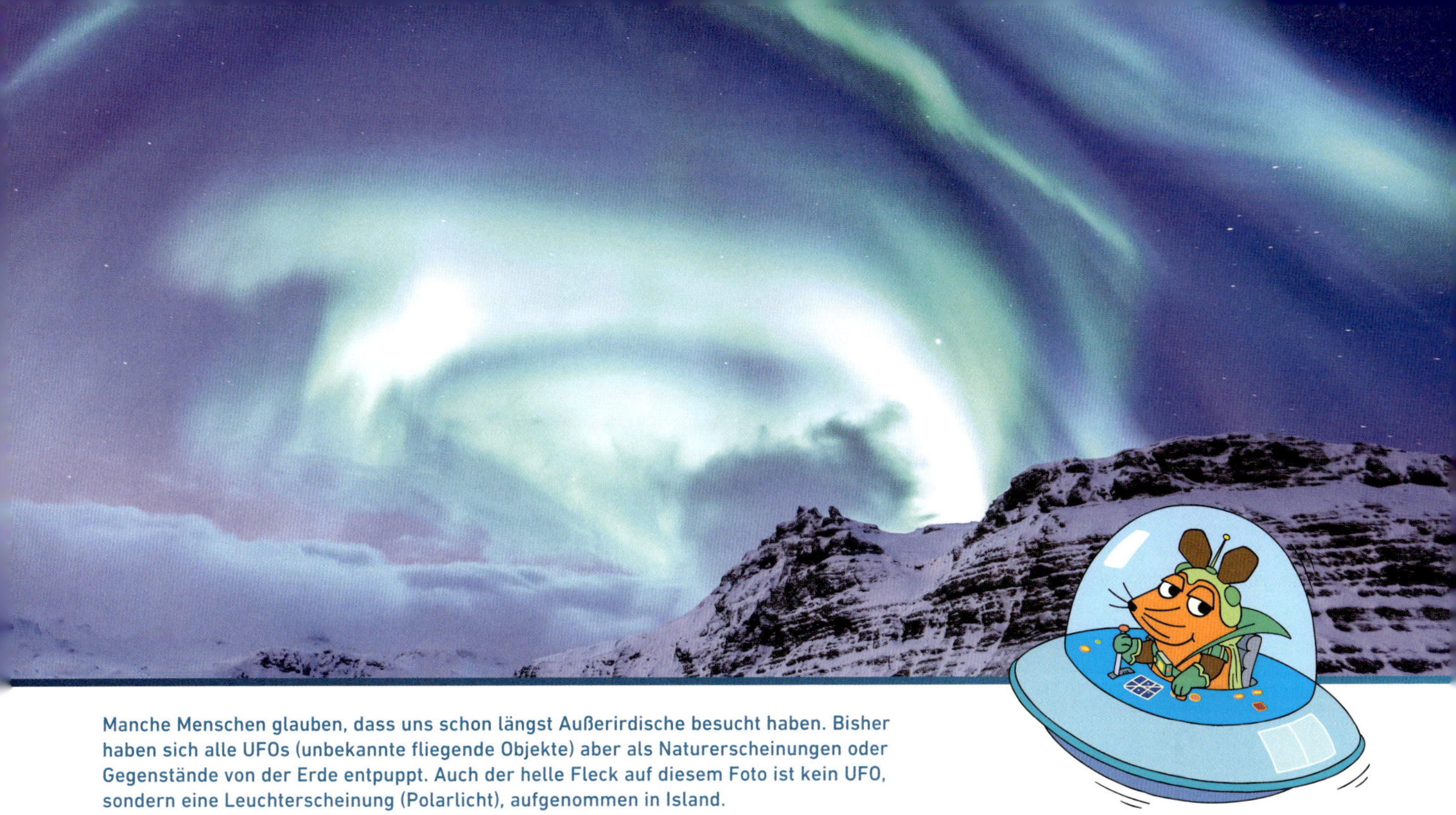

Manche Menschen glauben, dass uns schon längst Außerirdische besucht haben. Bisher haben sich alle UFOs (unbekannte fliegende Objekte) aber als Naturerscheinungen oder Gegenstände von der Erde entpuppt. Auch der helle Fleck auf diesem Foto ist kein UFO, sondern eine Leuchterscheinung (Polarlicht), aufgenommen in Island.

entstehen kann. Das Wichtigste: Es muss flüssiges Wasser geben und darf nicht zu heiß oder zu kalt sein.

Es wäre theoretisch möglich, dass es noch irgendwo Leben im All gibt. Vielleicht haben wir nur deshalb noch keinen Besuch bekommen, weil die anderen Wesen zu weit weg leben. Die Entfernungen im **Universum** sind unvorstellbar groß. Schon die Reise zu unserem Nachbarstern Proxima Centauri würde mit heutigen Raumschiffen 40.000 Jahre dauern.

Für den Fall, dass es wirklich Außerirdische gibt und sie uns Signale schicken, lauschen Wissenschaftler schon seit Jahren mit speziellen Geräten ins All.

Wenn eine **Raumsonde** in den Weltraum hinausfliegt, hat sie an Bord immer eine Tafel mit Grüßen und einigen wichtigen Informationen über uns Menschen.

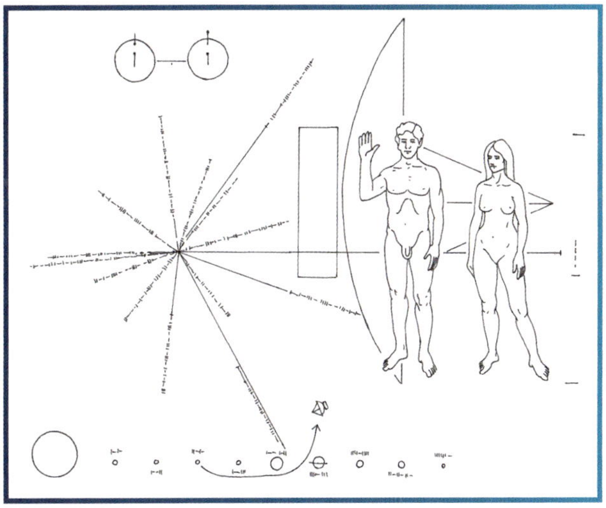

Auf der Tafel von Pioneer 10 sah man zum Beispiel, dass die Erde der dritte Planet der Sonne ist und wie die Körper von uns Menschen aussehen.

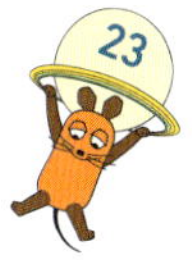

Wie sieht es auf dem Mars aus?

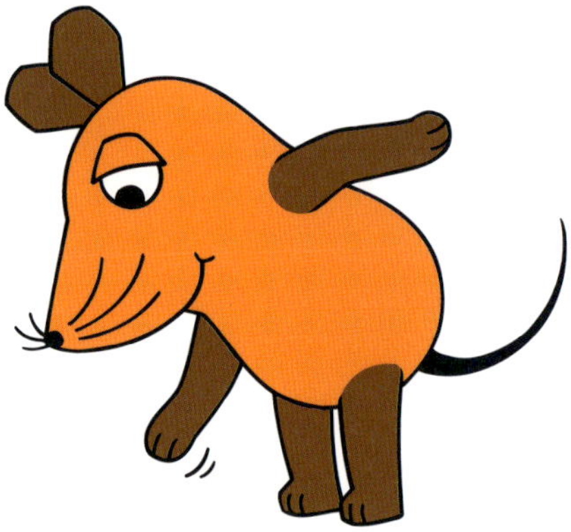

Im Jahr 1877 meinte der italienische Astronom Giovanni Schiaparelli, auf der Oberfläche des Mars seltsame Linien zu sehen. Vielleicht gibt es ja doch Marsmenschen?

Fast genau 100 Jahre später landeten die ersten **Raumsonden** auf dem Mars. Ihre Bilder zeigten Ebenen aus feinem rötlichen Sand, übersät mit Gesteinsbrocken, doch kein Leben weit und breit.

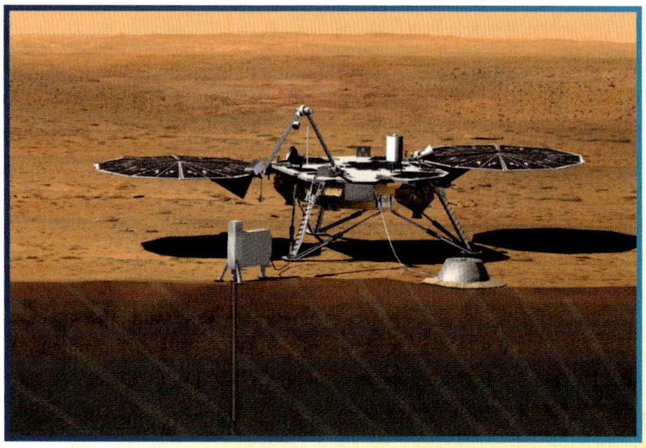

Raumsonden erkunden andere Planeten. Im Mai 2018 hat sich die US-Raumsonde „InSight“ auf den Weg zum Mars gemacht, um neue Informationen zu sammeln.

Du könntest auf dem Mars nicht atmen – der Planet hat nur eine ganz dünne Gashülle um sich herum. Sie besteht vor allem aus Kohlendioxid, einem Gas, das Menschen ausatmen. Außerdem ist es dort meist sehr kalt, nachts bis minus 120 Grad. Und es toben immer wieder gewaltige Staubstürme.

Ein Teil der Marsoberfläche besteht aus Ebenen und runden Kratern, die ähnlich aussehen wie die auf unserem Mond. Aber es gibt auch sehr tiefe Täler und erloschene Vulkane.

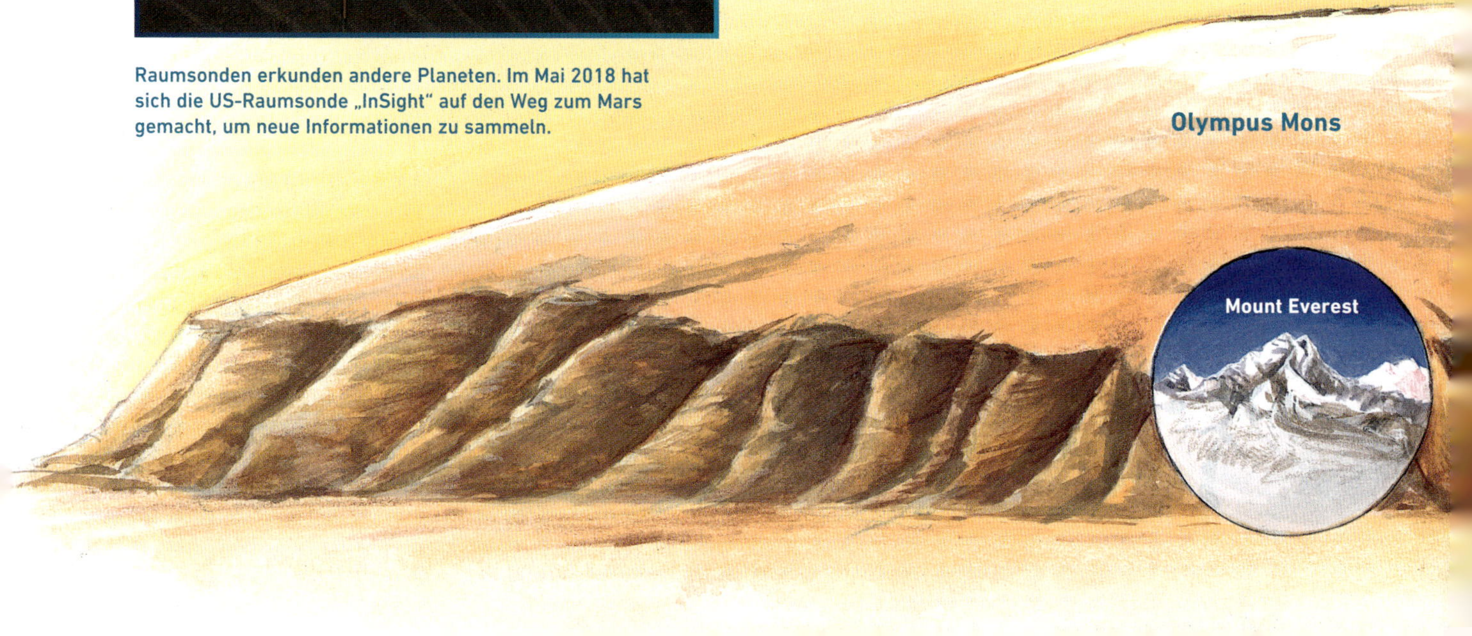

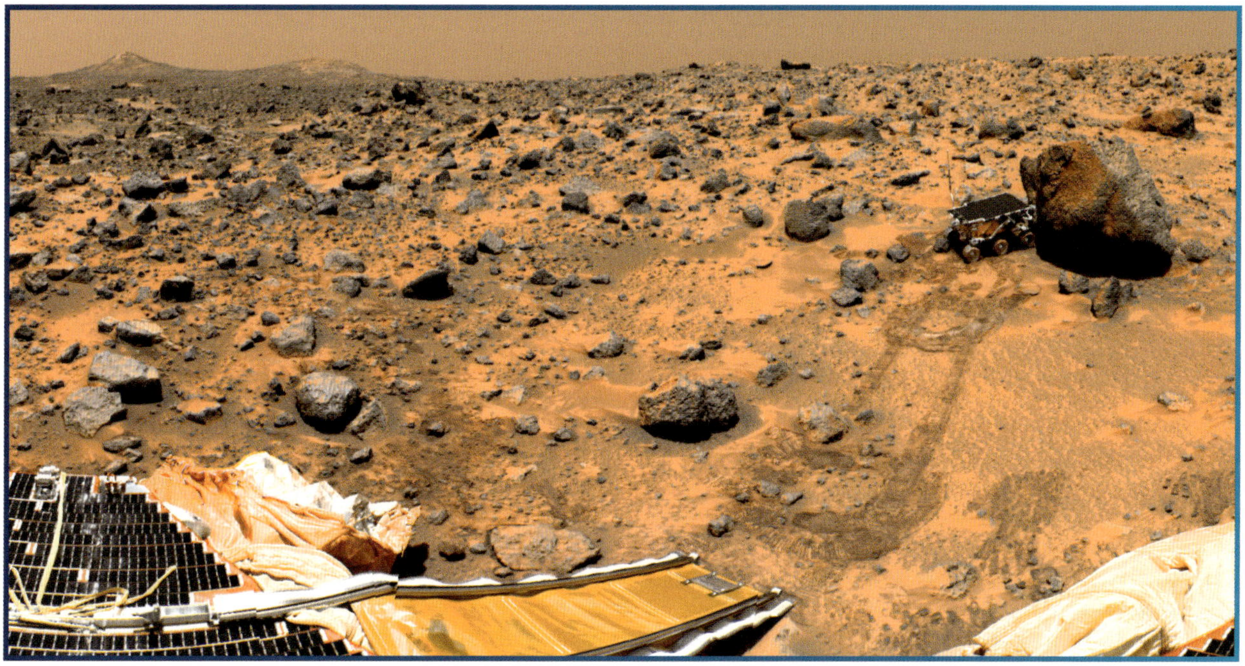

Die US-Raumsonde „Pathfinder“ (deutsch: Wegbereiter) hat 1997 besonders gute Bilder von der Marsoberfläche gemacht. Dafür hatte sie einen kleinen Roboter an Bord.

Vielleicht gab es auf dem Mars einmal Ozeane und Flüsse. Wahrscheinlich sind sie schon vor langer Zeit verdunstet. Aber Wasser ist auch heute noch auf dem Mars zu finden – zum Teil unter der Oberfläche, zum Teil als große Eisflächen an seinem Nord- und Südpol.

Der Mount Everest, der höchste Berg der Erde, ist 8.848 Meter hoch. Der Olympus Mons auf dem Mars ist 26.400 Meter hoch.

Die orangerote Farbe hat der Mars seinem eisenhaltigen Gestein zu verdanken: Die rote Farbe ist ganz einfach Rost!

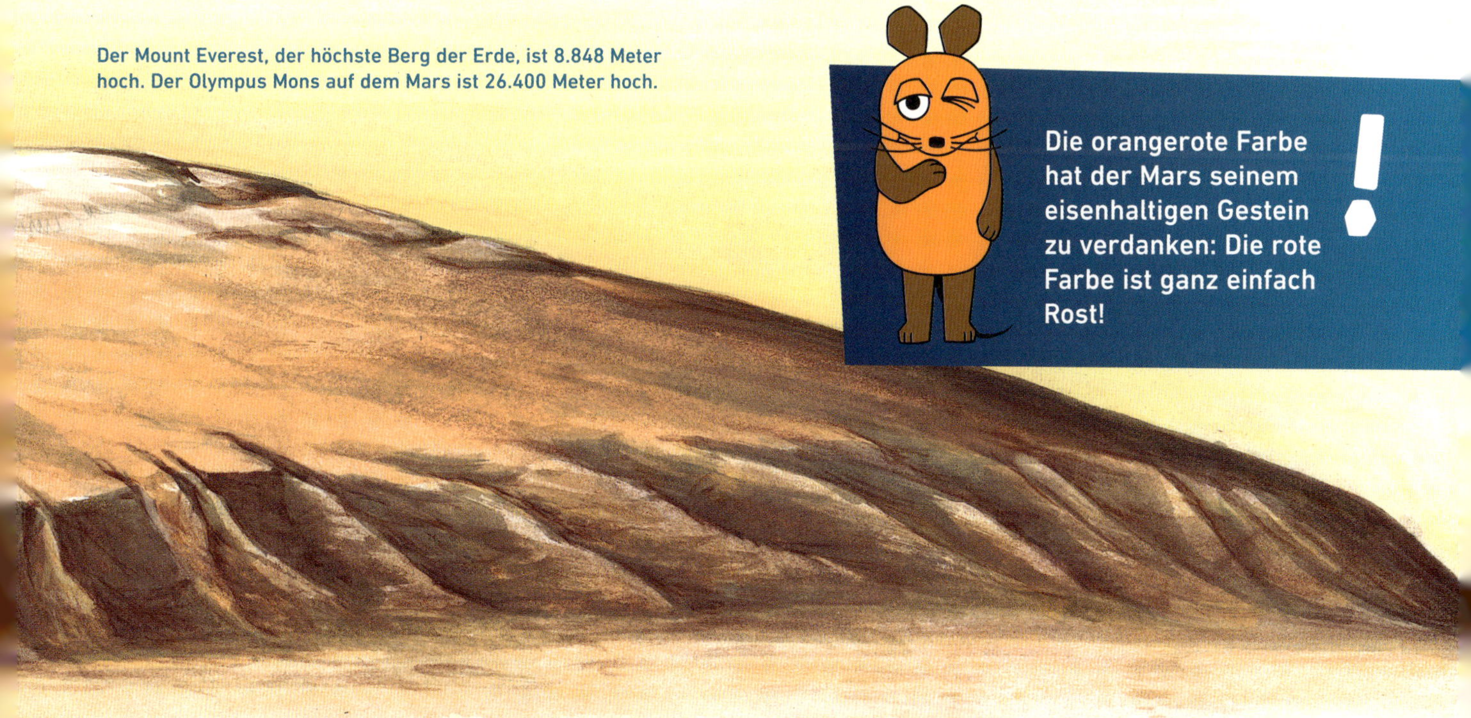

Kann man auf dem Jupiter spazieren gehen?

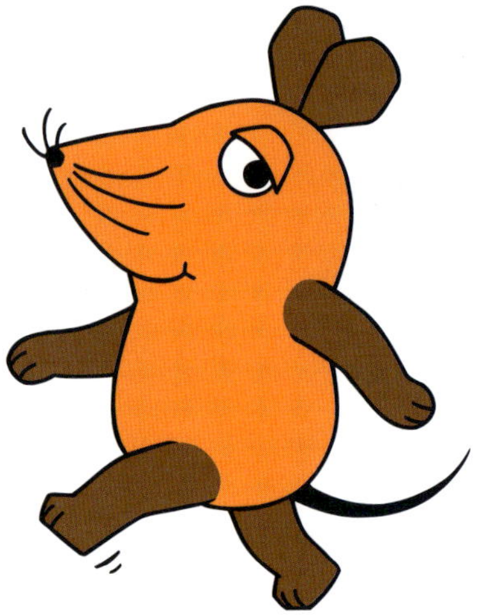

Auch mit einem Raumanzug wäre der Jupiter nicht fürs Wandern geeignet. Schon beim ersten Schritt würdest du tief einsinken.

Denn unter seinen Wolken ist kein fester Boden, sondern nur Gas. Irgendwann würdest du dann auf eine Schicht mit flüssigem Gas stoßen. Hier unten wäre schon so viel Gas über deinem Kopf, dass es mit riesigem Gewicht auf dich herunterdrücken würde.

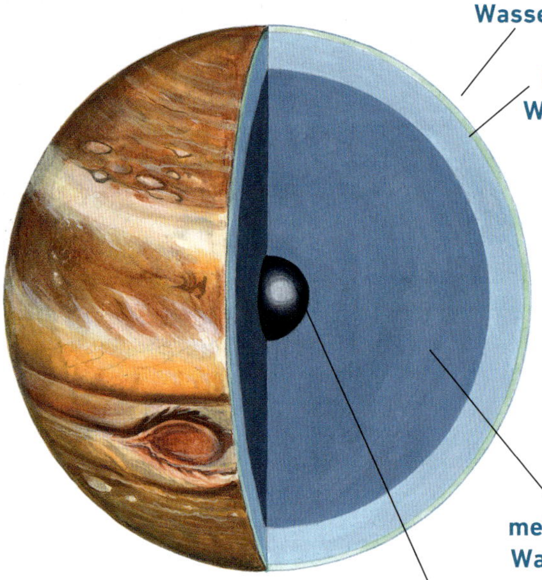

Das hält kein **Raumanzug** aus. Nach einer sehr langen Reise würdest du in der Mitte des Jupiters einen kleinen Kern aus Gestein und Eis finden.

Es gibt verschiedene Vermutungen, warum die äußeren Planeten unseres Sonnensystems aus Gas bestehen. Um das zu erklären, kannst du Folgendes ausprobieren: Wenn du bei starkem Wind steinige Gartenerde auf deine flache Hand legst, werden die leichten Teile weggeweht, die Steinchen bleiben liegen. Etwas Ähnliches ist wahrscheinlich passiert, als unser Sonnensystem noch eine wirbelnde Wolke aus Gas und Staub war. Auch damals gab es einen starken Wind: den **Sonnenwind**. Er bestand aus vielen Teilchen, die von der Sonne ausgesandt wurden.

Wahrscheinlich hat dieser Wind die Gase weggeschoben. Aus den leichten Stoffen bildeten sich die äußeren Planeten Jupiter, Saturn, Uranus und Neptun. Die festen, schweren Stoffe blieben in der Nähe der Sonne. Aus ihnen bildeten sich die inneren Planeten, die aus Gestein und Metallen bestehen.

Jupiter ist der Riese unter den Planeten des Sonnensystems; er ist so groß wie alle anderen zusammen.

Einzigartig ist er auch durch die bunten Wolkenbänder auf seiner Oberfläche. Mit einem einfachen Fernrohr kann man seinen Großen Roten Fleck sehen, einen gewaltigen Wirbelsturm, der schon seit Jahrhunderten tobt.

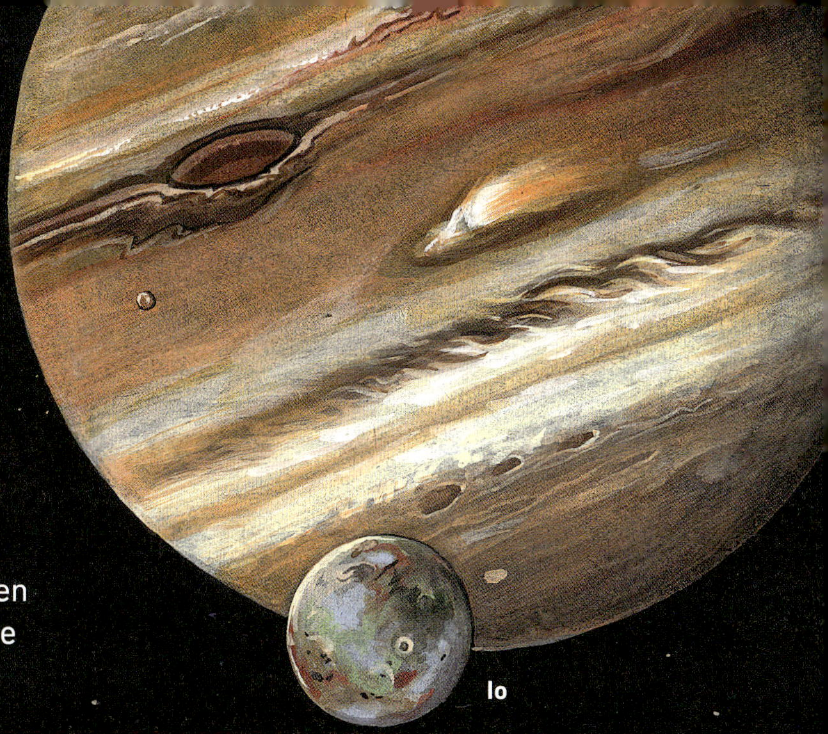

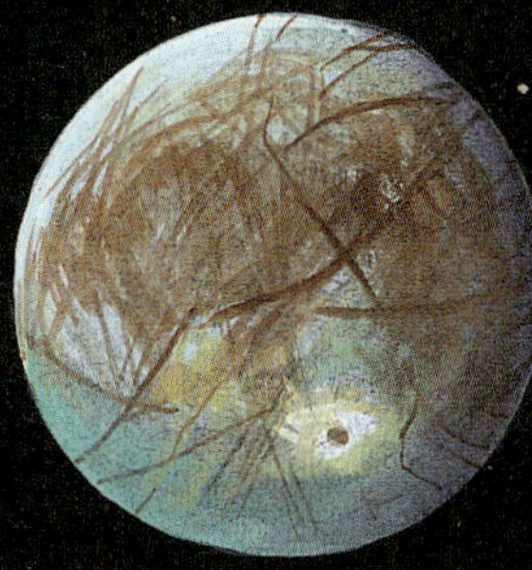

Der Jupiter wird von vielen großen Monden begleitet. Einer von ihnen heißt Europa.

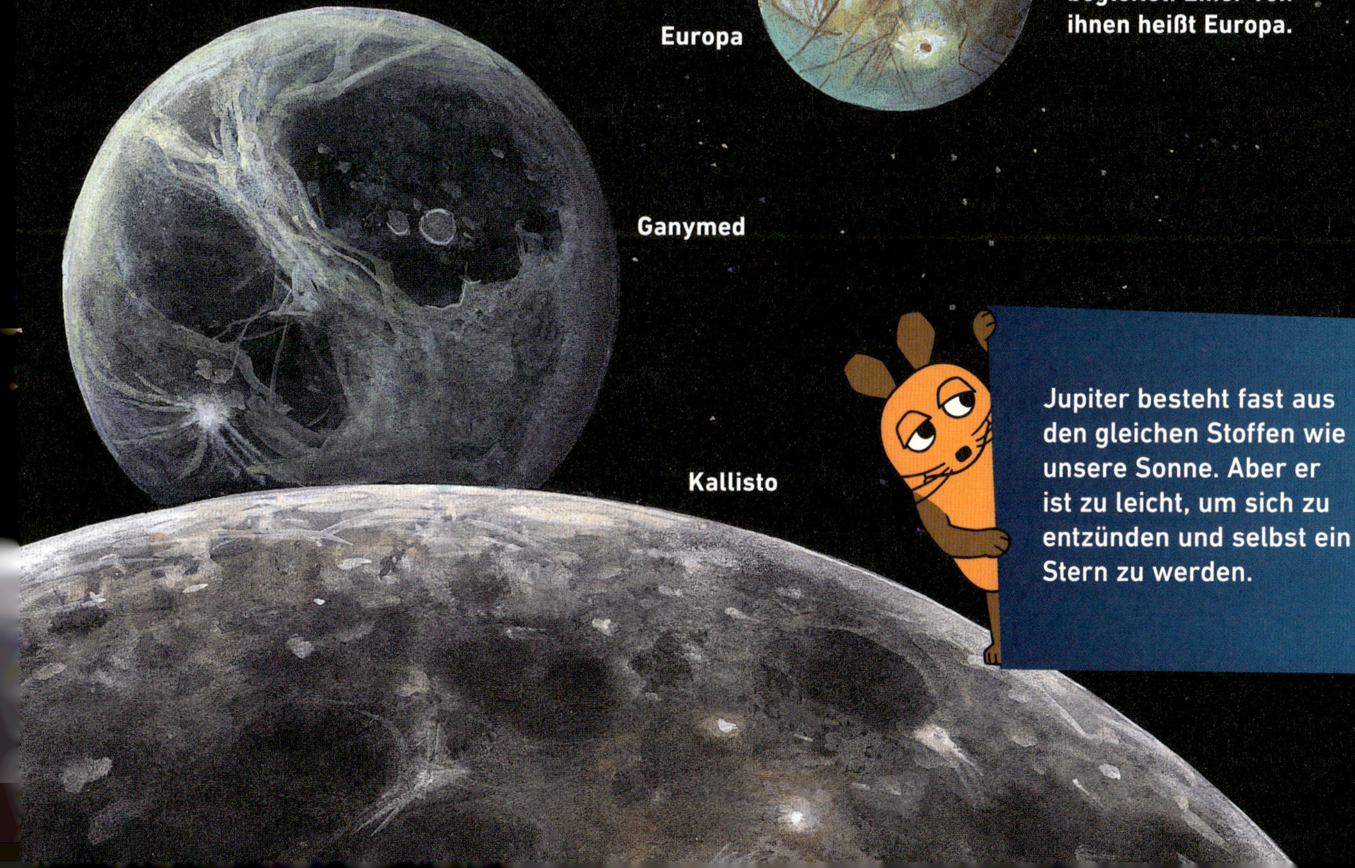

Jupiter besteht fast aus den gleichen Stoffen wie unsere Sonne. Aber er ist zu leicht, um sich zu entzünden und selbst ein Stern zu werden.

Warum hat der Saturn einen Ring?

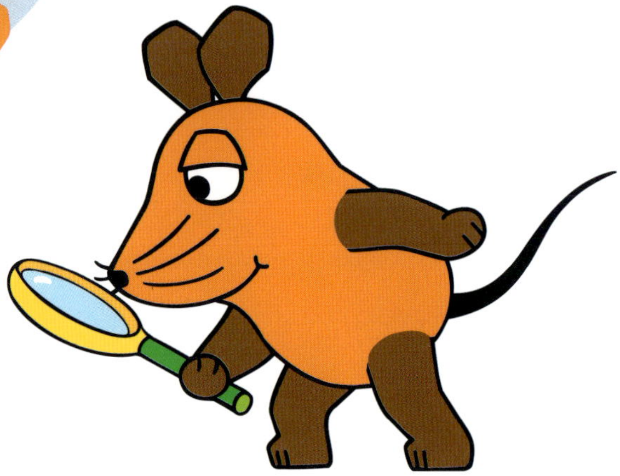

Der Saturn hat ganz viele Ringe. Wie der Planet zu diesen Ringen kam, können auch die Wissenschaftler nicht genau sagen. Doch sie haben ein paar Vermutungen.

Die Saturn-Ringe sind riesig, aber recht dünn. Ihre Dicke beträgt nur knapp hundert Meter. Sie bestehen aus vielen Eis- und Gesteinsklumpen. Manche sind so groß wie ein dreistöckiges Haus, die meisten aber so klein wie eine Erbse. All diese Brocken kreisen um den Saturn und bilden zusammen mehr als 100.000 einzelne Ringbänder.

Vermutung Nr. 1:

Manche Wissenschaftler nehmen an, dass die Ringe übrig geblieben sind, als Saturn entstanden ist. Planeten bilden sich aus kreisenden Gas- und Staubscheiben, die sich langsam unter der eigenen Schwerkraft zusammenziehen. Dadurch formt sich nach und nach ein Planet. Aus dem restlichen Material entstehen oft Monde – und bei großen Planeten manchmal auch Ringe.

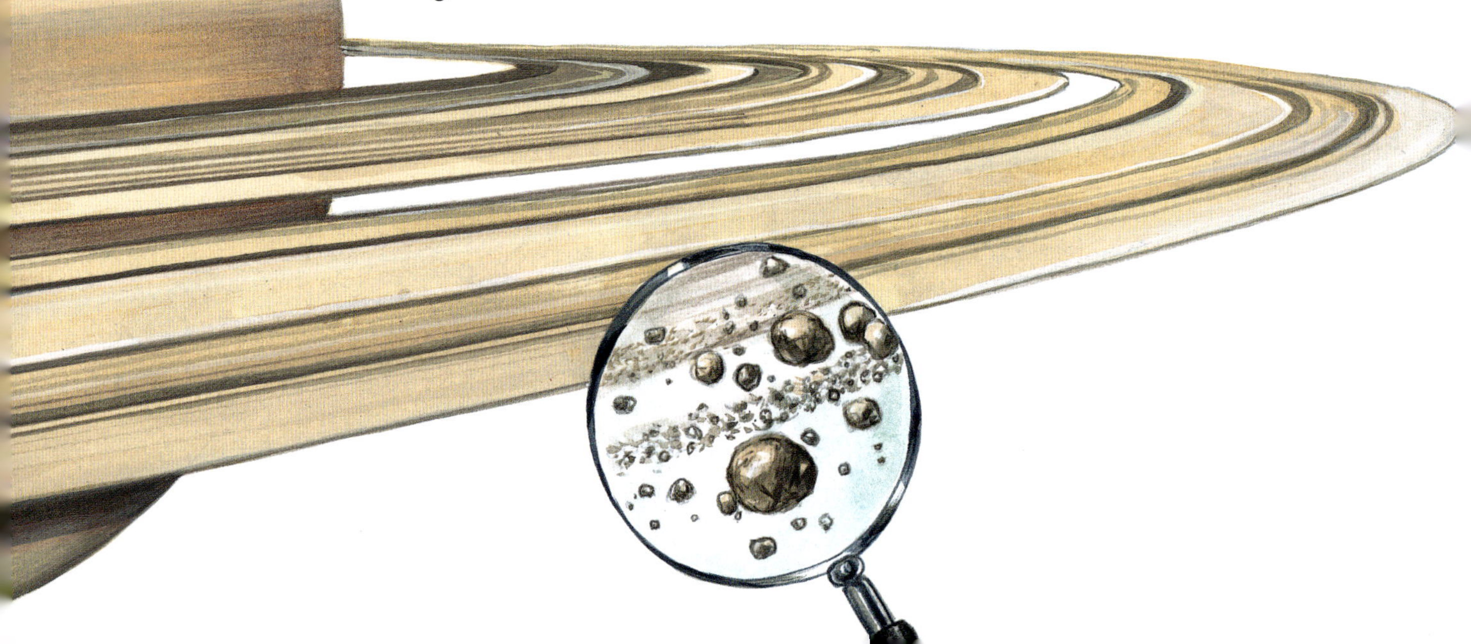

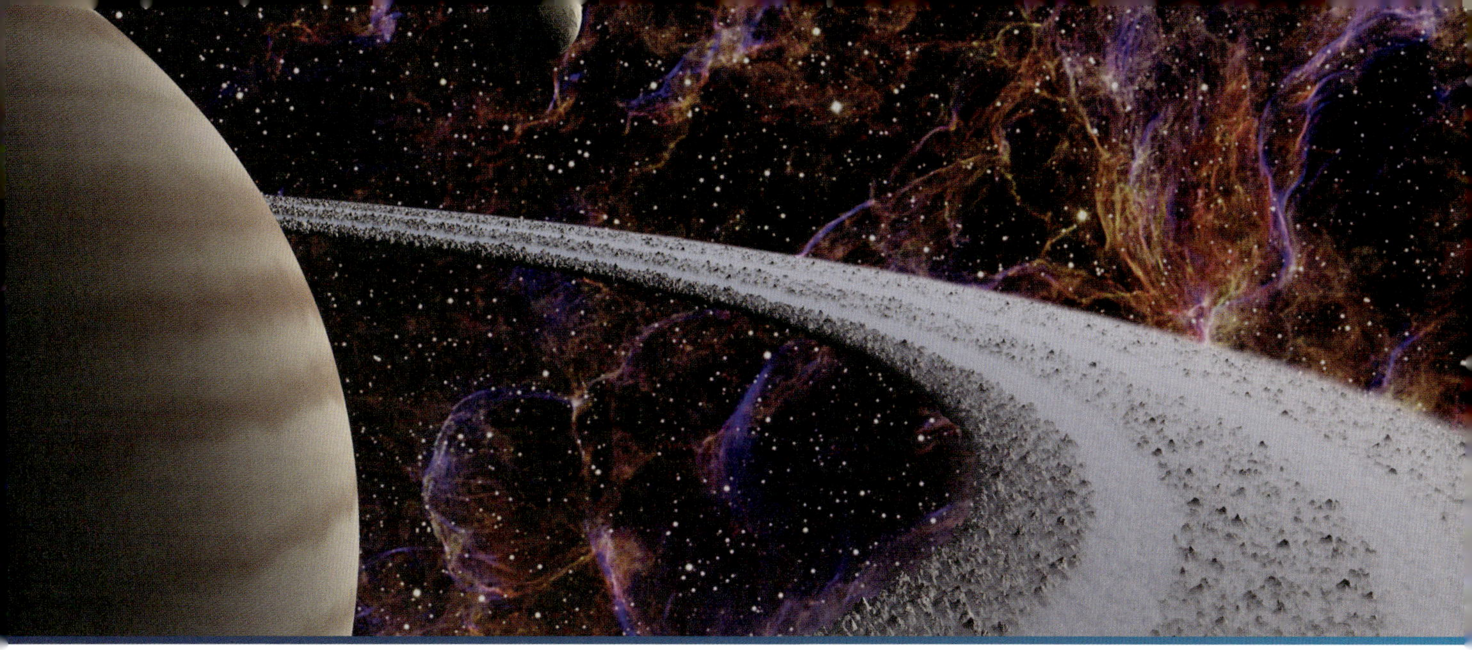

Vermutung Nr. 2:

Andere Wissenschaftler meinen, dass die Saturnringe viel später entstanden sind. Sie könnten Trümmer von Saturnmonden sein, die zusammengestoßen und zerbrochen sind. Die Brocken sind immer wieder zusammengestoßen und wurden so zu kleineren Körnchen zerrieben.

Übrigens haben auch die Planeten Jupiter, Neptun und Uranus Ringe. Aber sie sind kaum zu sehen und nicht so prächtig wie die des Saturn.

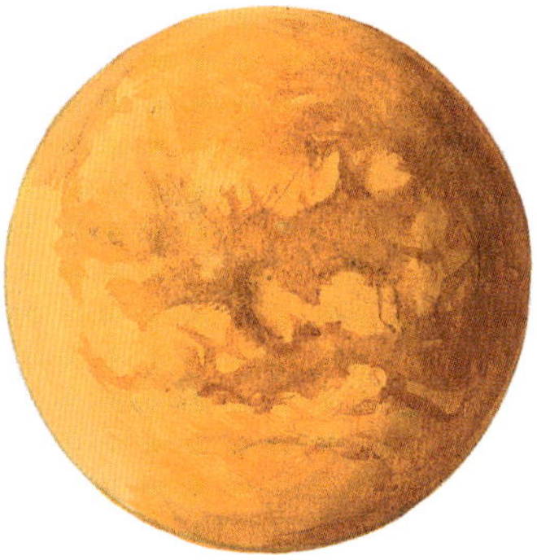

Titan
Größter Saturnmond. Er hat eine dichte Gashülle um sich herum, das ist für einen Mond sehr ungewöhnlich.

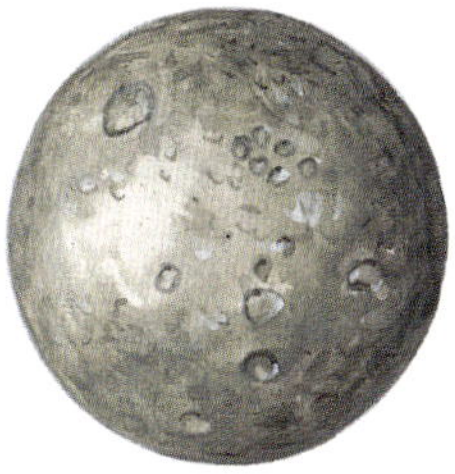

Rhea
Zweitgrößter Saturnmond. Er besteht zu zwei Dritteln aus Eis und zu einem Drittel aus Gestein.

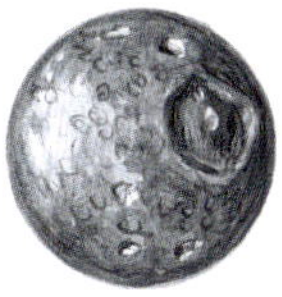

Mimas
Ein riesiger Krater verrät, dass Mimas einmal von einem großen Himmelskörper getroffen wurde.

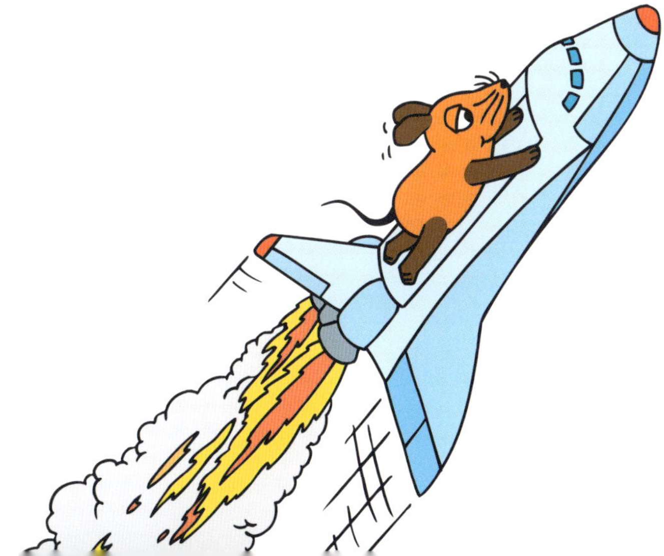

Woher kommen die Kometen?

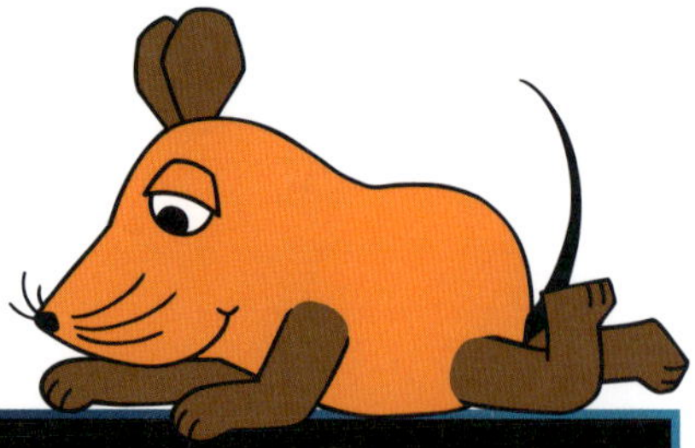

Kometen sind Klumpen aus Eis, Staub und gefrorenen Gasen. Wenn sie in der Nähe der Sonne vorbeifliegen, ziehen sie eine leuchtende Spur hinter sich her, die man deutlich am Himmel sehen kann. Früher hielt man Kometen für Unglücksboten, die schreckliche Ereignisse ankündigten.

Geheimnisvoll ist es, dass immer wieder neue Kometen auftauchen. Der Schlüssel zu diesem Rätsel ist die Bahn, auf der sie fliegen. Viele Kometen wandern aus fernen Weiten des Weltalls herbei, umrunden die Sonne, sodass man ihren Schweif am Himmel bewundern kann, und verschwinden dann. Manche für immer. Andere folgen einer Bahn, die sie regelmäßig in unsere Nähe führt. Der Komet **Halley** zum Beispiel kommt alle 76 Jahre in die Nähe der Sonne und ist dann bei uns am Himmel zu sehen (das nächste Mal im Jahr 2061).

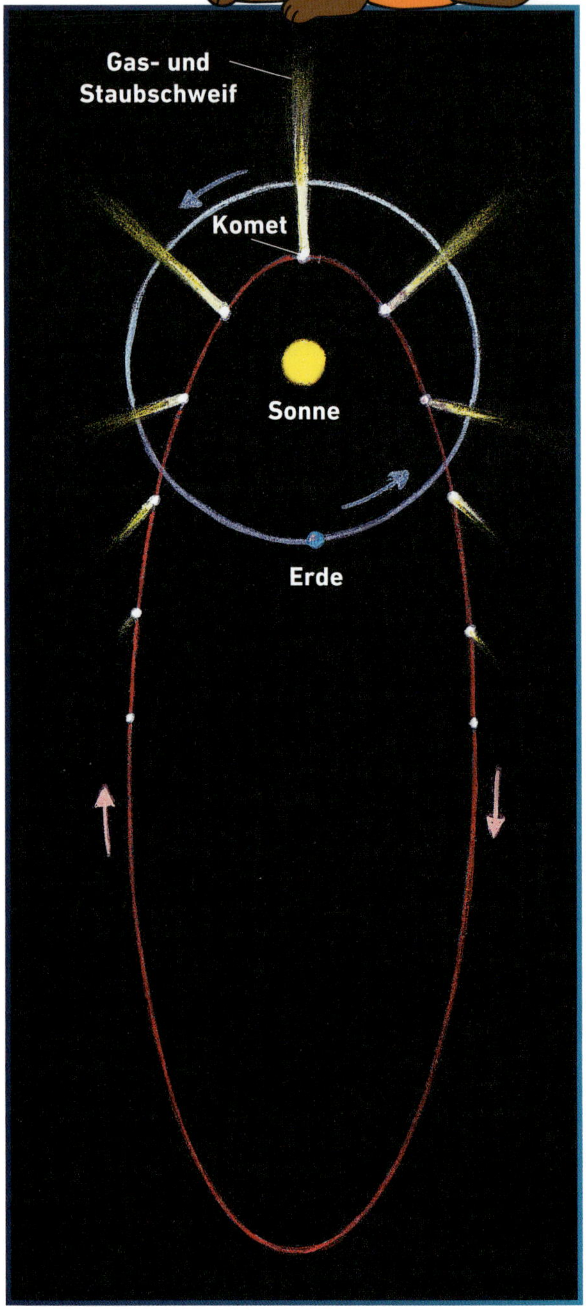

Wenn ein Komet in die Nähe der Sonne kommt, fängt seine Oberfläche an zu verdampfen – sein typischer Schweif aus Gas- und Staubteilchen entsteht und wird von der Sonne zum Leuchten gebracht.

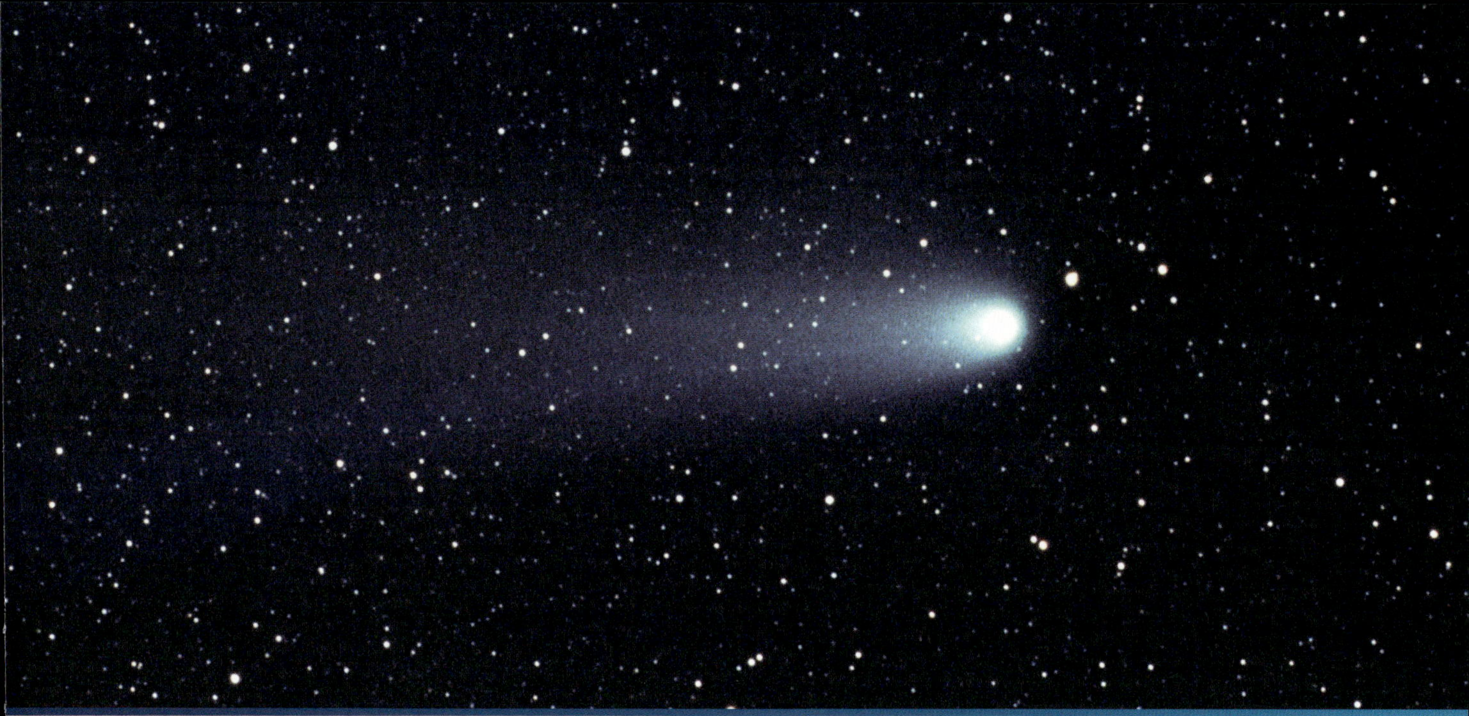

Das ist der Komet Halley. Sein Schweif kann sehr lang werden.

Forscher vermuten, dass Kometen wie Halley aus dem **Kuiper-Gürtel** stammen. So nennt man eine Gegend jenseits des Planeten Neptun, in der viele Eis- und Gesteinsbrocken die Sonne umkreisen. Ab und zu wird einer dieser Brocken aus seiner Bahn gerissen und wandert als Komet durch das Weltall.

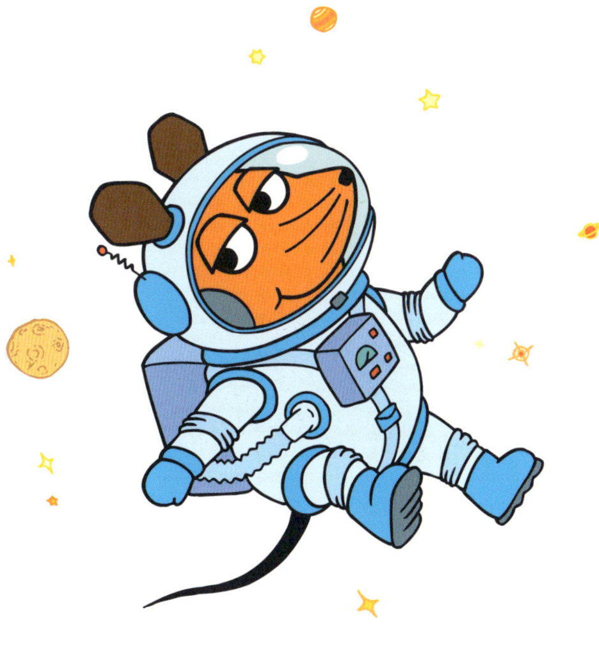

Kometen, die aus größerer Ferne stammen und nur alle paar tausend Jahre bei uns erscheinen, kommen wahrscheinlich aus der **Oortschen Wolke**. Forscher glauben, dass diese Wolke aus vielen Eisbrocken besteht und weit draußen das ganze **Sonnensystem** umgibt.

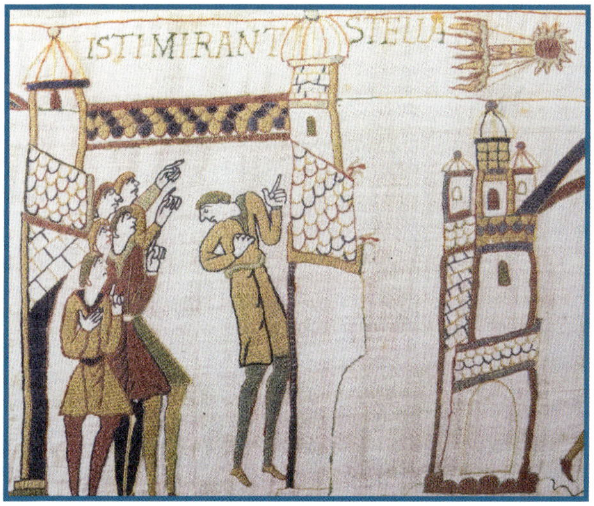

Den Kometen Halley kennen die Menschen schon seit sehr langer Zeit, weil man ihn ohne Fernrohr sehen kann. Hier ist er auf einem Wandteppich aus dem 11. Jahrhundert abgebildet.

Warum fallen manchmal so viele Sternschnuppen?

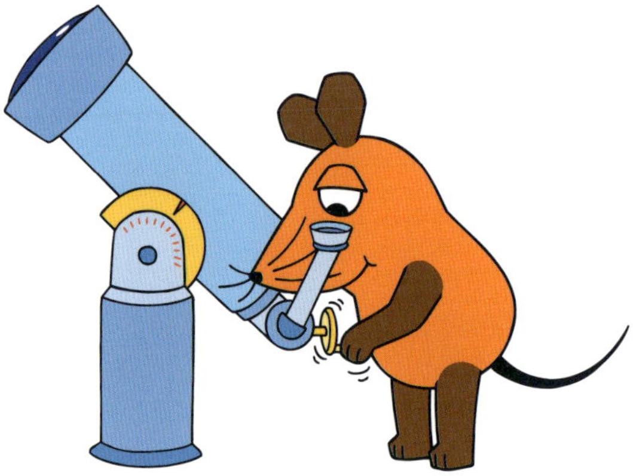

In manchen Nächten saust eine Sternschnuppe nach der anderen über den Himmel. Das hängt mit den Kometen zusammen.

Sternschnuppen entstehen aus Gesteinstrümmern, die durchs Weltall wandern. Oft sind sie nicht größer als ein Kieselstein. Wenn solche Krümel auf die Lufthülle der Erde prallen, überstehen sie das nicht.

Sie bewegen sich hundertmal schneller als eine Pistolenkugel. Dadurch reiben die Luftteilchen sehr stark über ihre Oberfläche. Das heizt die Steinchen so sehr auf, dass sie schon hoch über dem Erdboden verbrennen. Das sehen wir

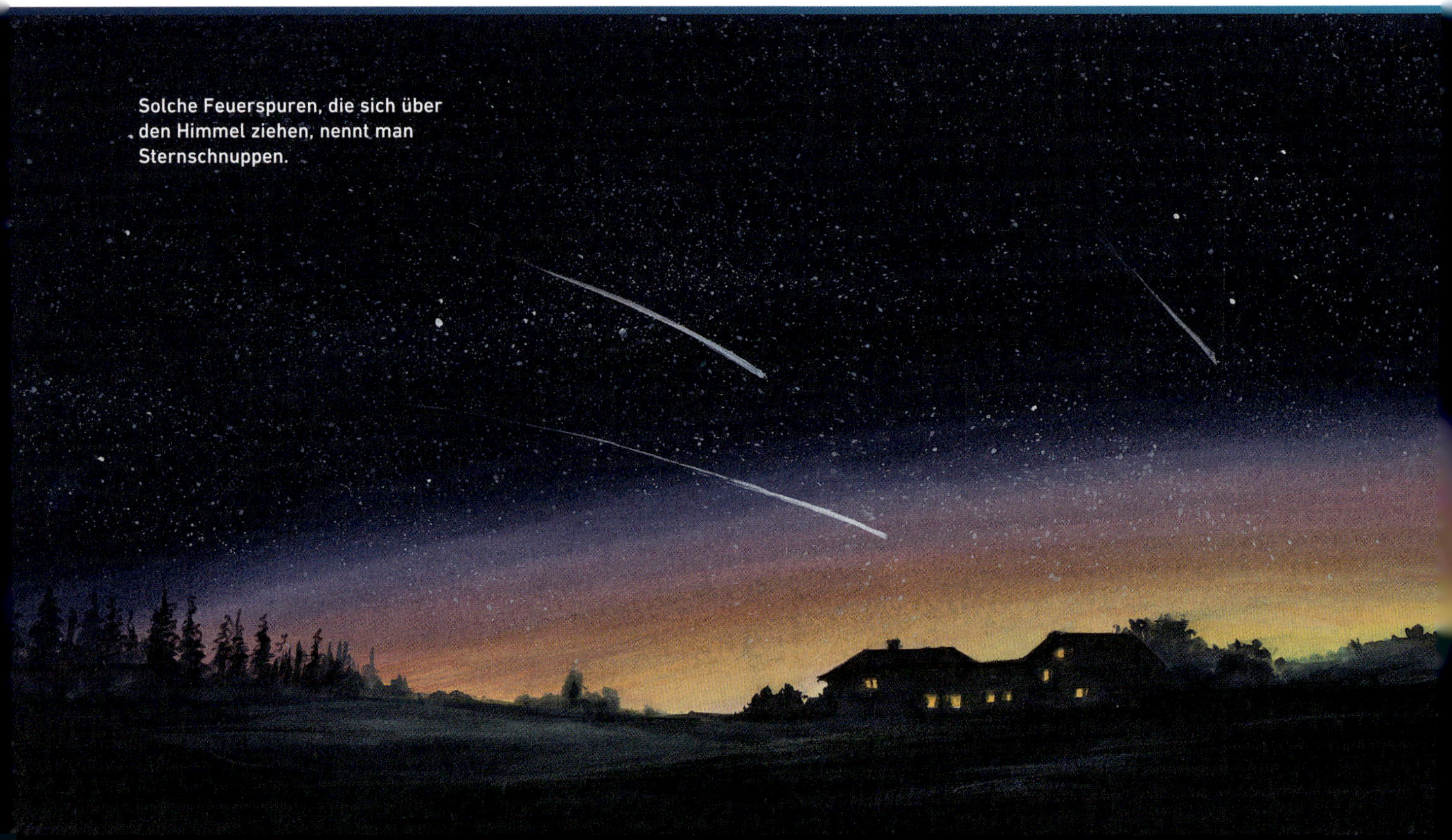

Solche Feuerspuren, die sich über den Himmel ziehen, nennt man Sternschnuppen.

als flammende Spur am Himmel. Ein paarmal im Jahr treffen besonders viele solcher Teilchen auf die Erde. Und das hängt mit den Kometen zusammen:

Stell dir vor, du gehst mit dreckigen Schuhen durch die Wohnung. Dabei hinterlässt du eine Spur von Erdkrümeln und Steinchen. Kometen hinterlassen ähnliche Spuren im Weltall. Jedes Mal, wenn sie an der Sonne vorbeifliegen, schmilzt etwas vom Eis und löst sich zusammen mit Gestein und Staub von dem Kometen. Wenn die Erde auf ihrem Weg um die Sonne in so eine Kometendreck-Spur gelangt, gibt es nachts ein hübsches Feuerwerk zu bewundern!

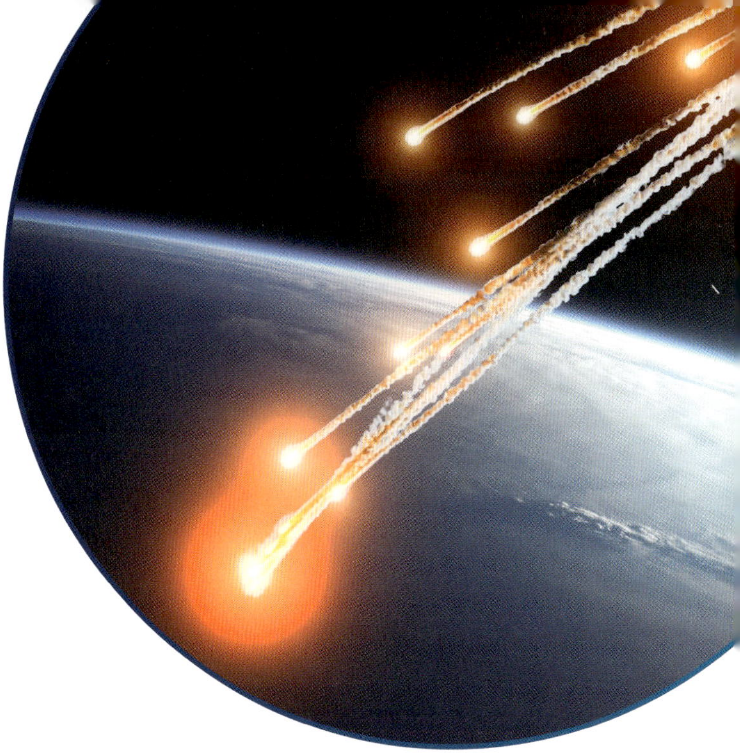

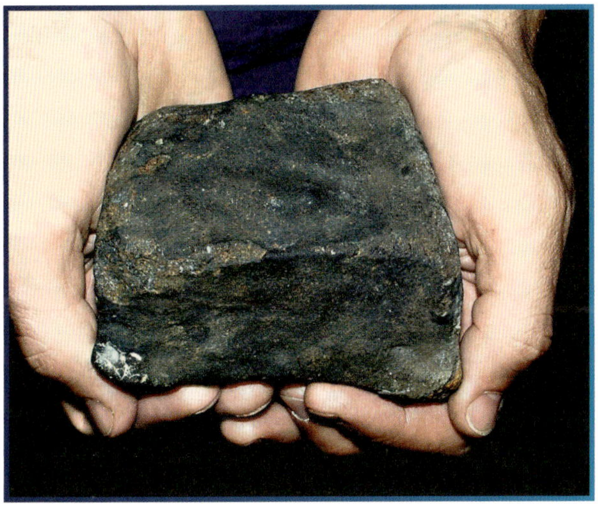

Ein etwa 20 Kilo schwerer Meteorit landete im Jahr 2002 in der Nähe des berühmten Schlosses Neuschwanstein. Vom Neuschwanstein-Meteoriten hat man schon mehrere Bruchstücke gefunden. Dieses hier ist 1,7 Kilo schwer.

Viele Sternschnuppen und **Meteore** gibt es jedes Jahr

- im Sternbild Löwe am 17. November, verursacht vom Kometen Tempel-Tuttle.
- im Sternbild Perseus vom 11. – 14. August, verursacht vom Kometen Swift-Tuttle.
- im Sternbild Zwillinge vom 7. – 17. Dezember, verursacht vom Himmelskörper Phaeton.

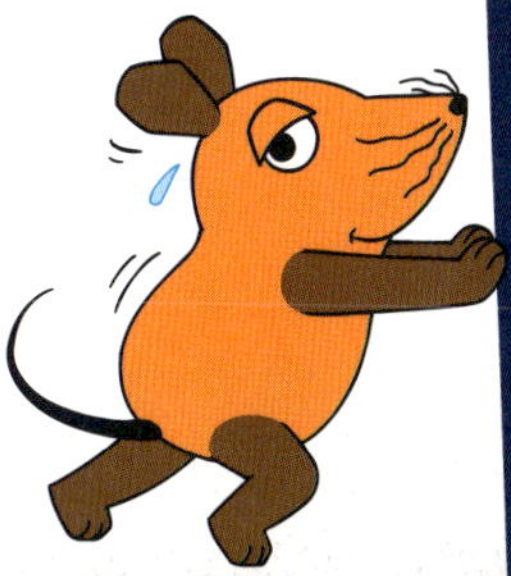

Größere Brocken aus dem Weltall verbrennen oft nicht ganz. Rund 20.000 sogenannter Meteorite regnen pro Jahr auf die Erde herab. !

Wer hat sich die Sternbilder ausgedacht?

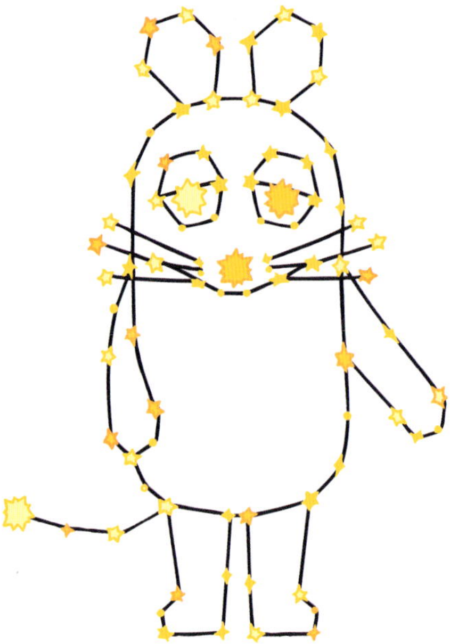

Wenn du zum Himmel hochschaust, kannst du in klaren Nächten die Sterne über uns sehen. Sie alle scheinen sich im Laufe der Nacht langsam zu bewegen, weil sich die Erde dreht. Aber sie bleiben immer am selben Platz.

Man kann diese einzelnen Leuchtpunkte zu verschiedenen Bildern verbinden. Die ältesten Sternbilder, die wir heute noch kennen, bekamen vor etwa 3.500 Jahren von den Babyloniern ihre Namen.

Sie erfanden die zwölf Sternbilder, die der „Tierkreis“ genannt werden. Später, vor etwa 2.000 Jahren, griffen die Menschen in Griechenland diese Bilder auf. In dem alten Sternbild „Löwe“ sahen sie das Tier,

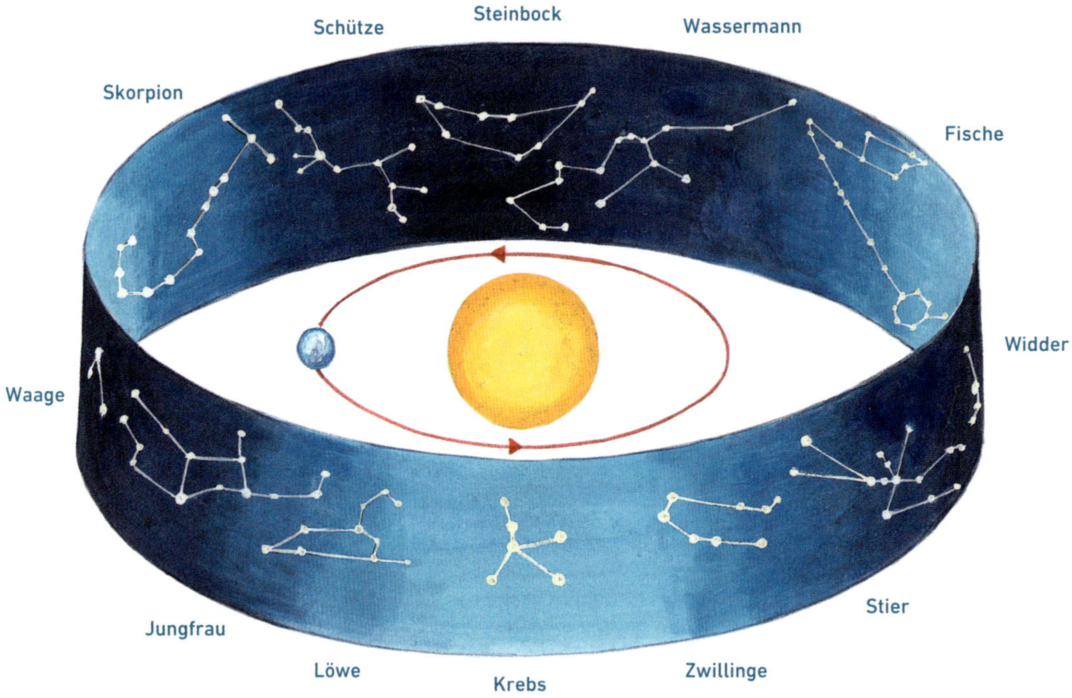

Die zwölf Tierkreiszeichen liegen alle auf einer Bahn, auf der die Sonne scheinbar über den Himmel zieht.

das ganze Städte verwüstete, bis der Held Herakles es besiegte. Sie dachten sich noch viele andere Sternbilder aus. Zum Beispiel tauften sie eines „Orion“ nach einem starken Jäger aus einer ihrer Sagen.

Durch die Bahn der Erde um die Sonne verändern die Sternbilder mit den Jahreszeiten ihre Lage am Himmel.

Doch die Griechen konnten nur die Sternbilder benennen, die sie bei sich auf der nördlichen Erdhalbkugel am Himmel sahen. Von der Südhalbkugel, zum Beispiel von Australien aus, sieht man einen ganz anderen Sternenhimmel.

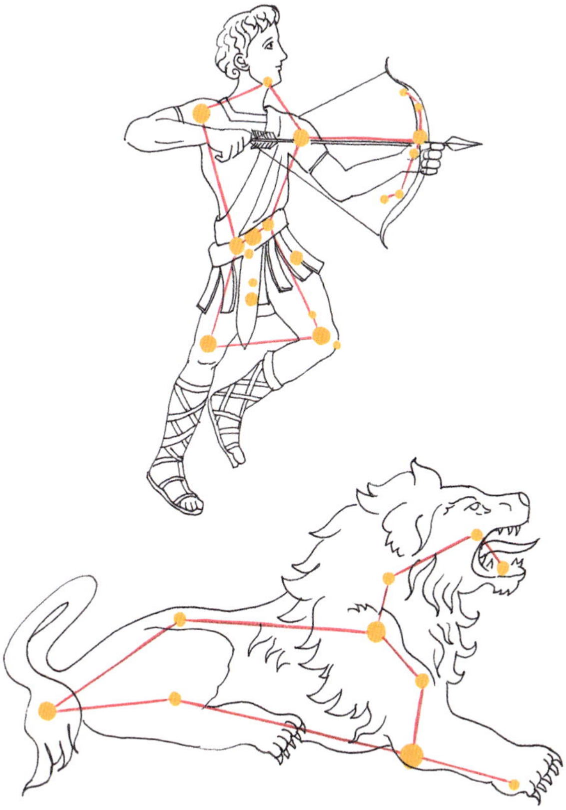

So kann man sich „Orion“ und den „Löwen“ vorstellen. Das Sternbild Orion ist im Winter besonders gut zu sehen, der Löwe im Frühjahr.

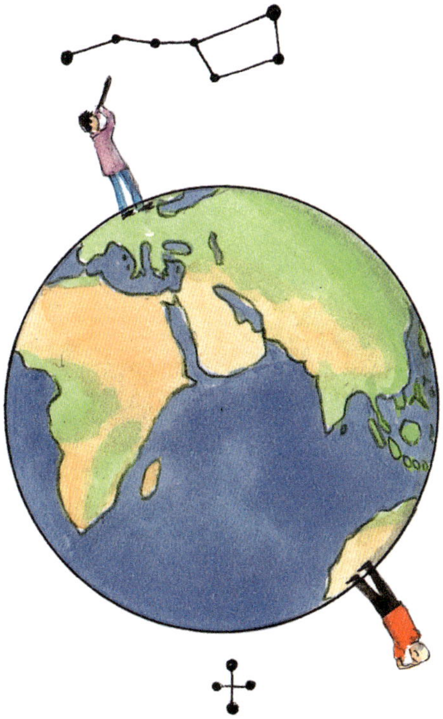

Auf der nördlichen Hälfte der Erde sieht man das Sternbild „Großer Wagen“, auf der südlichen Hälfte das „Kreuz des Südens“. Diese Sternbilder nutzten die Seefahrer schon früher, um sich zu orientieren.

Astronomen machten sich vor 400 Jahren daran, neue Sternbilder zu erfinden, zum Beispiel „Giraffe“ oder „Einhorn“. Auch technische Erfindungen wie das „Mikroskop“ wurden am Himmel verewigt. Es gibt sogar ein Sternbild namens „Luftpumpe“.

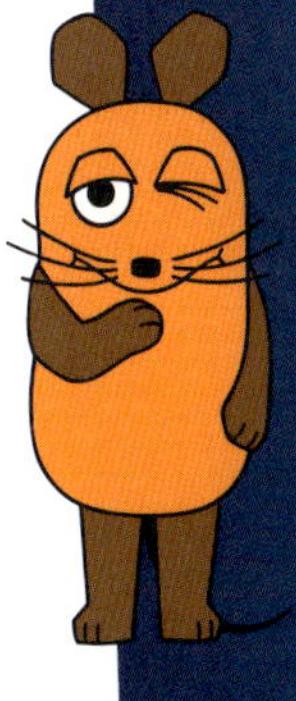

Die Sterne eines Sternbilds haben meist nichts miteinander zu tun und liegen oft sehr weit voneinander entfernt. Nur von uns aus sieht es so aus, als würden sie Muster bilden.

Wie laut war der Urknall?

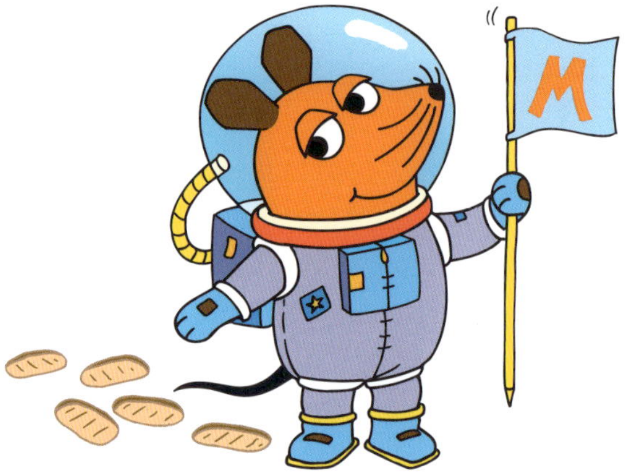

Noch weiß man nicht genau, wie unser Universum entstanden ist. Es gibt aber Beweise dafür, dass alles mit einem Urknall angefangen hat – der größten Explosion, die es je gab.

Man könnte meinen, dass der Urknall unglaublich laut war. Doch tatsächlich konnte man den Urknall gar nicht hören. Denn man kann ein Geräusch nur hören, wenn Luft da ist, die **Schallwellen** weiterleiten kann. Im Weltraum gibt es aber keine Luft, dort ist es immer ganz still.

Weil beim Urknall vor 13,7 Milliarden Jahren niemand dabei war, können wir nur vermuten, was genau passiert ist. Bisher nehmen die Wissenschaftler an, dass am Anfang ein unvorstellbar kleiner Punkt im Nichts anfing, sich auszudehnen. Daraus entstand das gigantische **Universum**, wie wir es heute kennen.

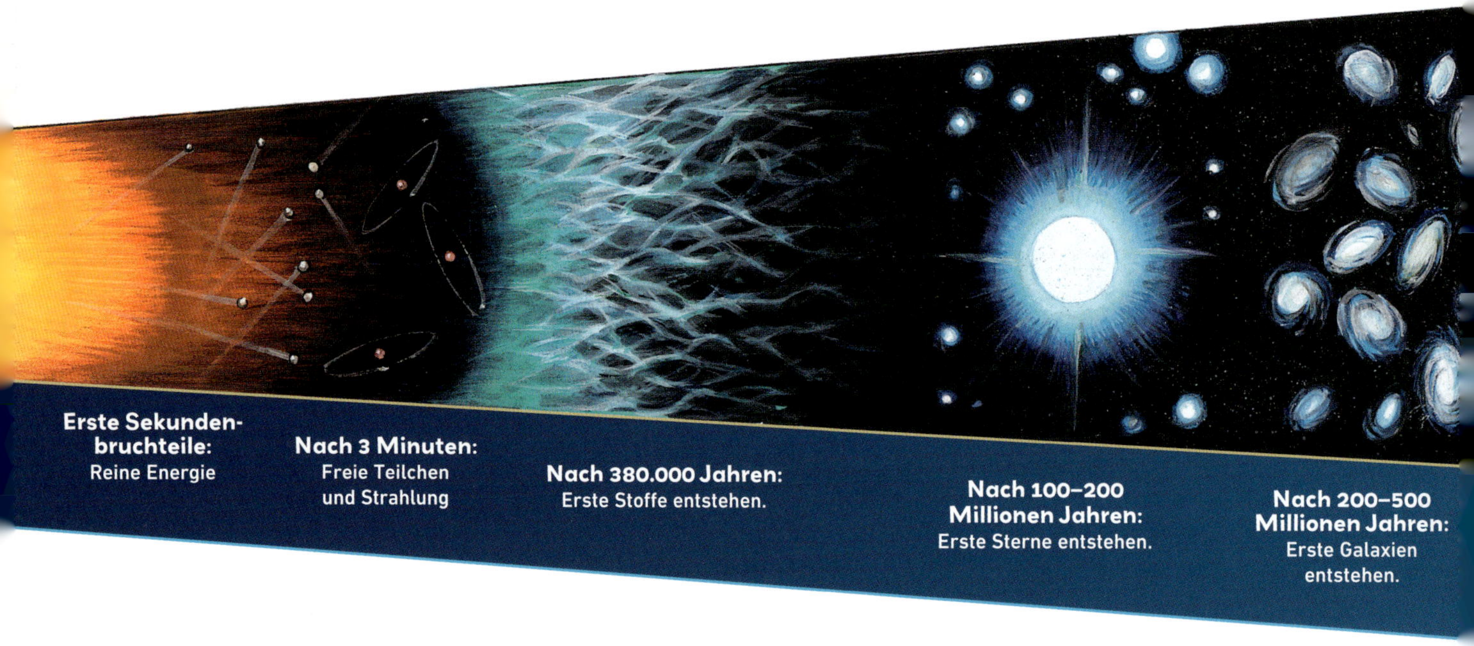

Erste Sekundenbruchteile: Reine Energie
Nach 3 Minuten: Freie Teilchen und Strahlung
Nach 380.000 Jahren: Erste Stoffe entstehen.
Nach 100–200 Millionen Jahren: Erste Sterne entstehen.
Nach 200–500 Millionen Jahren: Erste Galaxien entstehen.

In den ersten Sekundenbruchteilen herrschten wahrscheinlich unglaublich hohe Temperaturen. Als das Universum größer und kühler wurde, verwandelte sich die Energie des Urknalls in eine heiße Suppe aus Teilchen und Strahlung. Erst nach etwa 380.000 Jahren war das Weltall so weit abgekühlt, dass sich die ersten Stoffe, wie es sie heute gibt, bilden konnten. Es waren einfache Gase. Diese Gase waren im Weltraum nicht gleichmäßig verteilt. Gaswolken bildeten sich und in ihnen ballten sich Klumpen zusammen. In diesen Klumpen wurde es nach etwa 100 bis 200 Millionen Jahre so dicht und heiß, dass sie sich entzündeten: So entstanden die ersten **Sterne**. Diese waren riesig groß und explodierten bald, dabei schleuderten sie ihr Material in den Weltraum. Daraus bildeten sich kleinere, länger brennende Sterne wie unsere Sonne.

!

Das Universum hat sich seit dem Urknall sehr stark ausgedehnt und wird immer noch größer. Das weiß man, weil alle weit entfernten Galaxien von uns wegfliegen. Wohin sich das Universum ausdehnt, ist noch ein Rätsel!

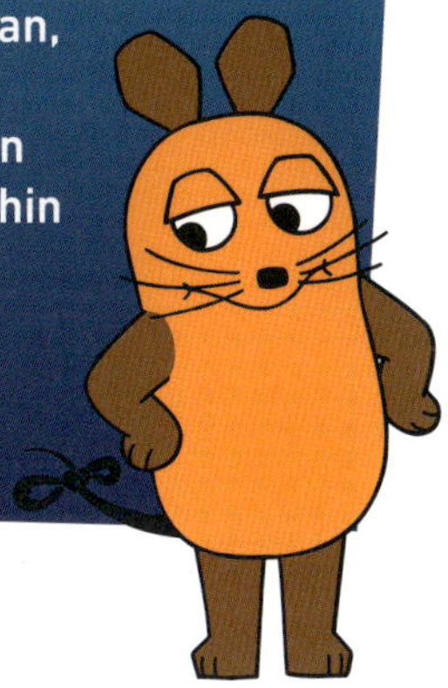

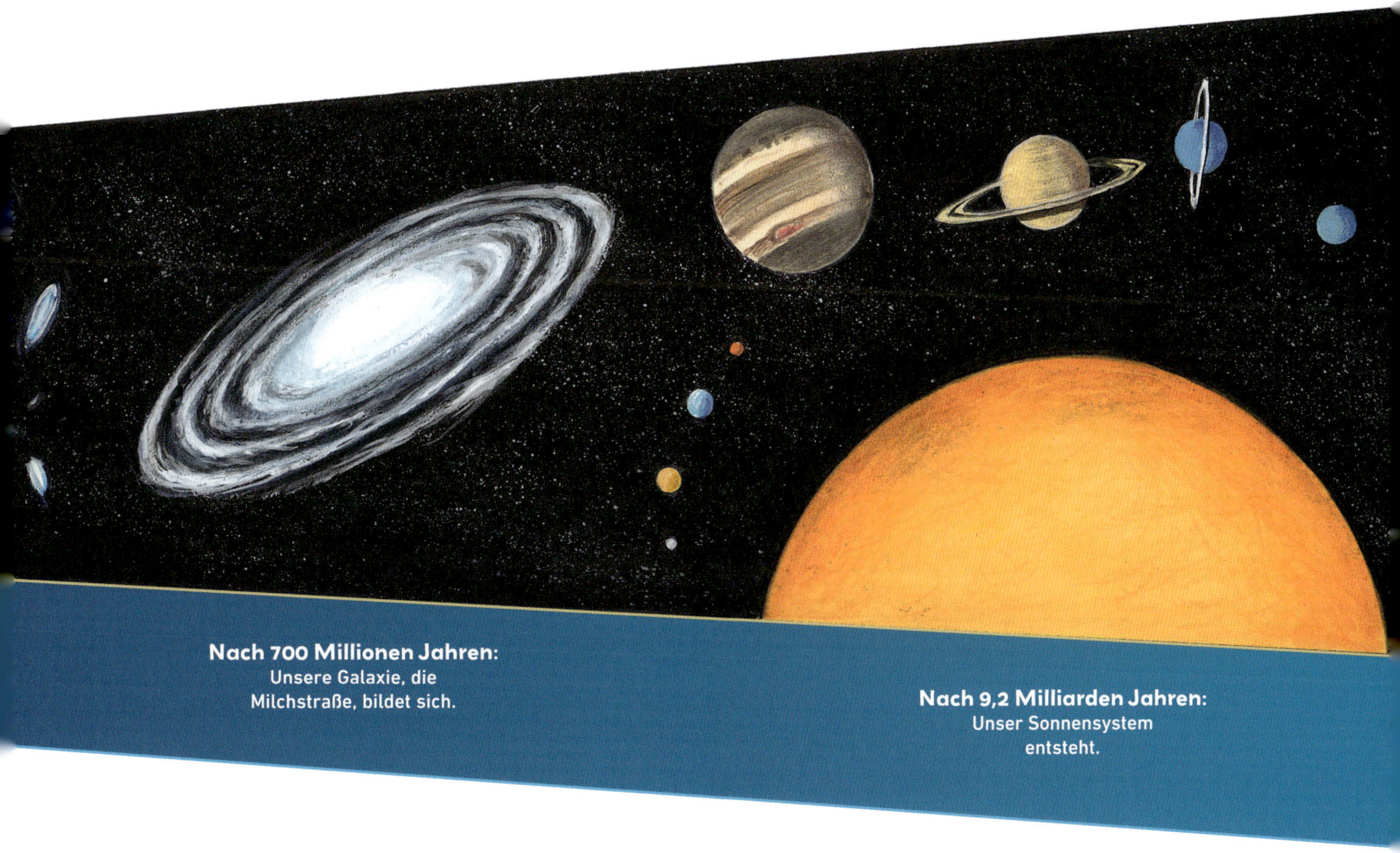

Nach 700 Millionen Jahren:
Unsere Galaxie, die Milchstraße, bildet sich.

Nach 9,2 Milliarden Jahren:
Unser Sonnensystem entsteht.

Warum leuchten die Sterne?

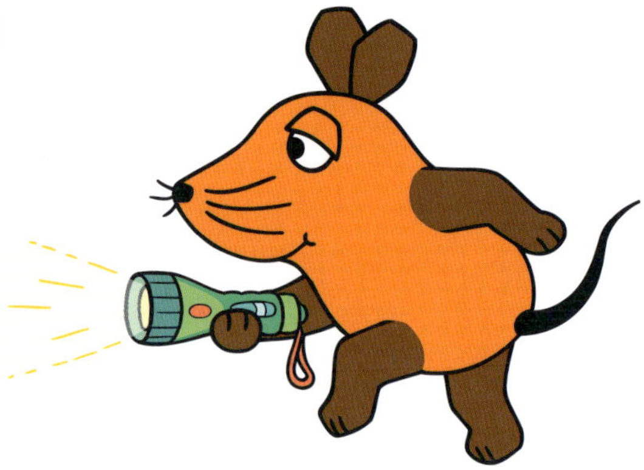

Sterne sind glühende Kugeln aus Gas. Und alles, was glüht, sendet Hitze und Licht aus. Dieses Licht sehen wir als Leuchtpunkte am Himmel.

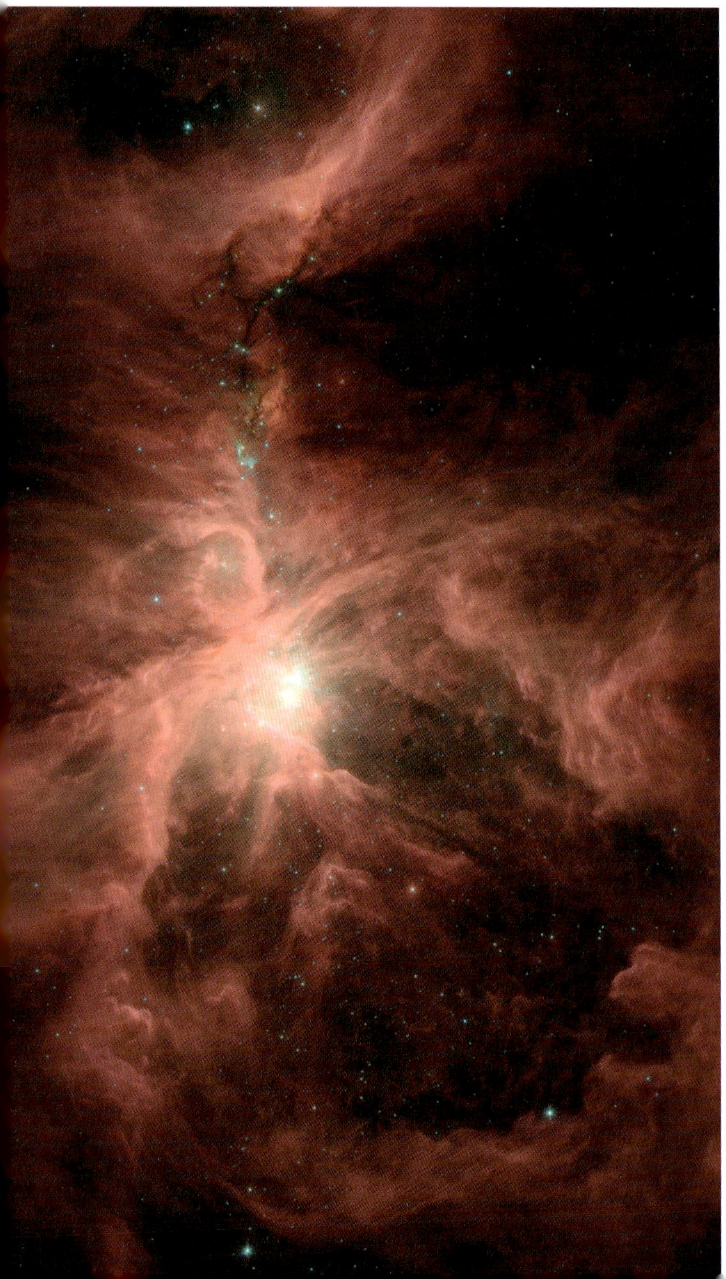

Junge Sterne entstehen aus Gaswolken. Manchmal, wenn ein alter Stern explodiert, gehen Druckwellen durchs All. Diese Wellen drücken Gaswolken in ihrer Nähe zusammen. An manchen Stellen bilden sich Klumpen. Durch ihre eigene Schwerkraft ziehen sich diese Klumpen zu riesigen Gasbällen zusammen.

Jetzt sind die neuen Sterne schon fast fertig, aber sie leuchten noch nicht. Wenn ein Gasball sehr groß und schwer geworden ist, werden die Teilchen in seinem Inneren zusammengedrückt. Immer zwei Teilchen verschmelzen zu einem einzigen, größeren. Dabei wird enorm viel Energie frei und der neue Stern beginnt von selbst zu glühen und damit auch zu leuchten.

Sterne können in unterschiedlichen Farben leuchten. Durch ein Teleskop kann man das von der Erde aus gut sehen: Junge Sterne sind meist bläulich-weiß, Sterne mittleren Alters gelb und ältere Sterne rot (oder weiß, dann nennt man sie „Weißer Zwerg“).

Hier, im Orion-Nebel, werden gerade neue Sterne geboren.

Wenn der Gasklumpen zu klein war, um sich selbst zu entzünden, wird er manchmal zu einem „Braunen Zwerg“. Diese leuchten nur ganz schwach.
Sterne können unterschiedlich groß sein. Im Vergleich zu einem **Weißen Zwerg** ist unsere Sonne riesig. Neben dem größten Stern, den man bisher entdeckt hat, würde sie winzig aussehen. Dieser Stern, ein „Roter Überriese“, ist etwa 2.000-mal so groß wie unsere Sonne.

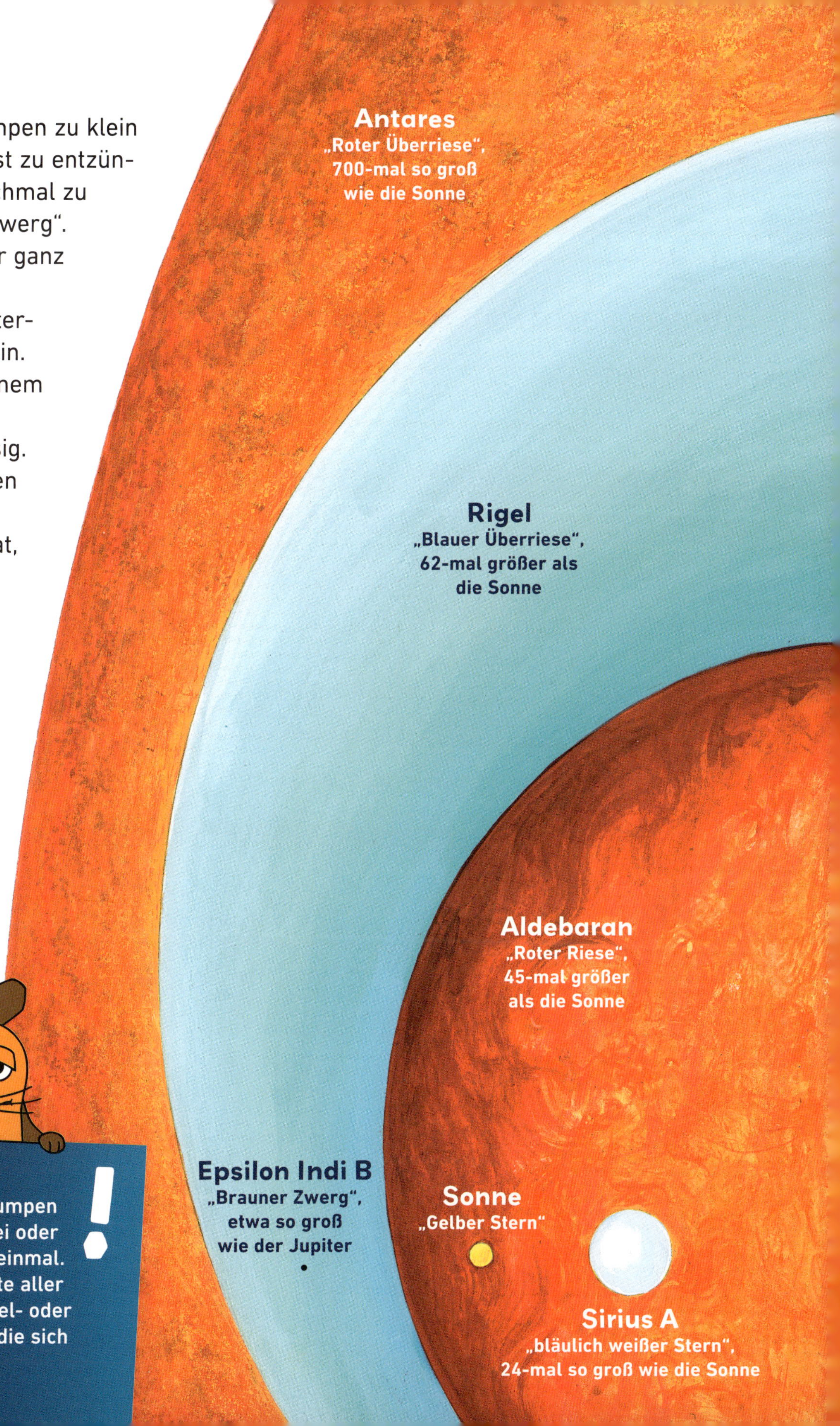
Antares
„Roter Überriese“, 700-mal so groß wie die Sonne
Rigel
„Blauer Überriese“, 62-mal größer als die Sonne
Aldebaran
„Roter Riese“, 45-mal größer als die Sonne
Epsilon Indi B
„Brauner Zwerg“, etwa so groß wie der Jupiter
Sonne
„Gelber Stern“
Sirius A
„bläulich weißer Stern“, 24-mal so groß wie die Sonne

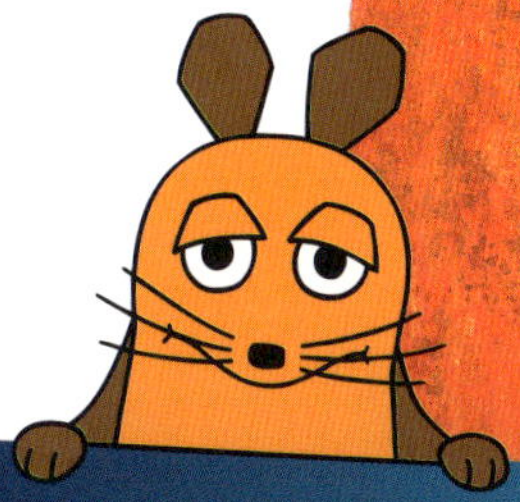

!

Aus einem Gasklumpen entstehen oft zwei oder mehr Sterne auf einmal. Mehr als die Hälfte aller Sterne sind Doppel- oder Mehrfachsterne, die sich umkreisen.

Können Sterne sterben?

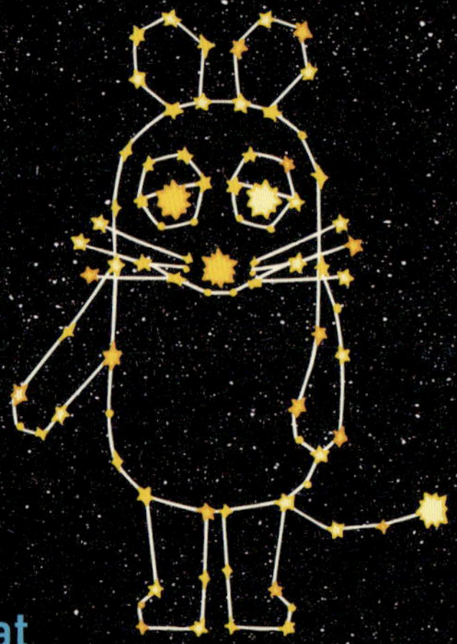

Auch Sterne leben nicht ewig. Wie lange sie strahlen, hängt davon ab, wann ihnen das Gas, das als Brennstoff dient, ausgeht. Auch unsere Sonne verbrennt Gas. Sie hat ihren Gasvorrat aber erst zur Hälfte verbraucht. Sie wird wohl noch sechs Milliarden Jahre lang leuchten.

Sterne, die größer, schwerer und heißer sind als unsere Sonne, verbrauchen ihren Brennstoff sehr viel schneller. Schon nach einer Million Jahre wird ihr Brennstoff knapp. Dann beginnen sie andere Stoffe in ihrem Inneren zu verbrennen. Das gibt ihnen einen Energieschub: Sie blähen sich auf und werden zu einem immer größer werdenden „Roten Riesen“.

Wenn ihre letzten Brennstoffe verbraucht sind, platzen die Sterne in einer gewaltigen Explosion auseinander. Das nennt man **Supernova**.

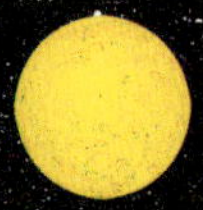

großer
gelber Stern

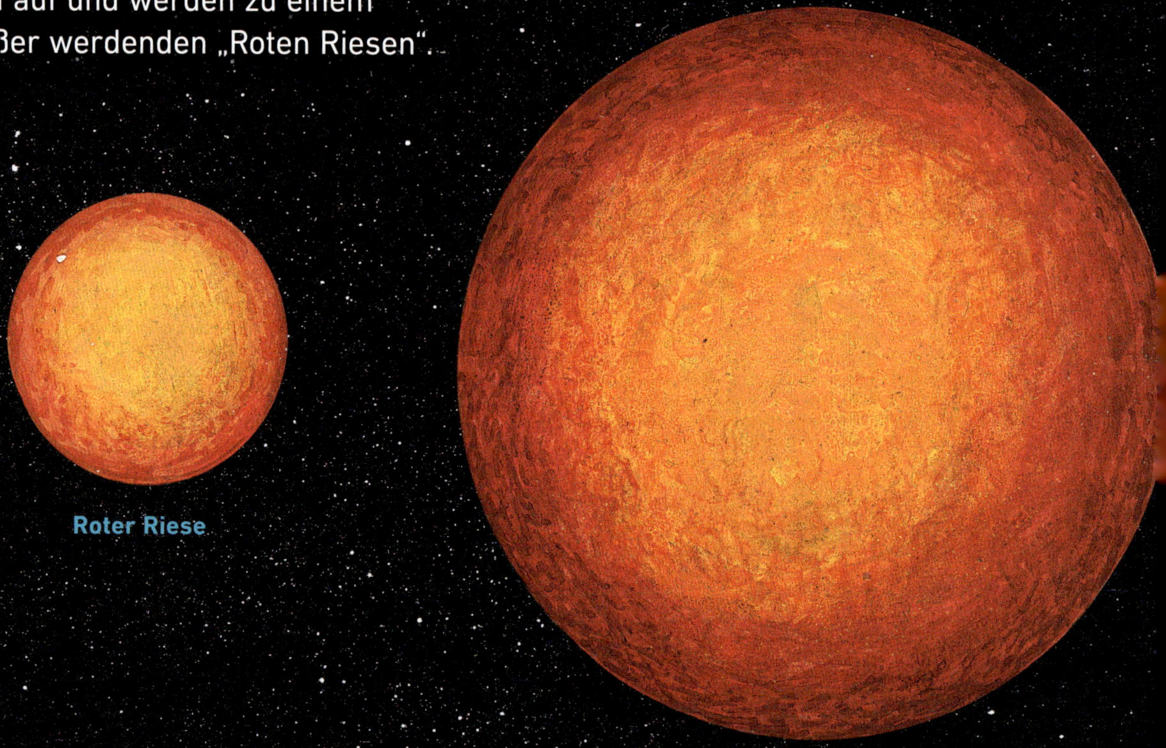

Roter Riese

Roter Überriese

Danach bleibt nicht viel von dem Stern übrig. Er schrumpft oft zu einem Neutronenstern zusammen.

Bei besonders großen und schweren Sternen ist die Schwerkraft so stark, dass sie am Ende in sich selbst zusammenstürzen. Es bleibt fast nichts mehr von ihnen übrig. Nur ein Schwarzes Loch, ein fast unsichtbarer Himmelskörper, der den Forschern noch viele Rätsel aufgibt.

Auch ein kleiner Stern bläht sich nach mehreren Milliarden Jahren zu einem Roten Riesen auf. Doch er explodiert nicht, sondern fällt in sich zusammen. Er ist ab jetzt ein Weißer Zwerg, ein Stern, der kaum größer ist als die Erde. Er wird immer kühler und erlischt schließlich.

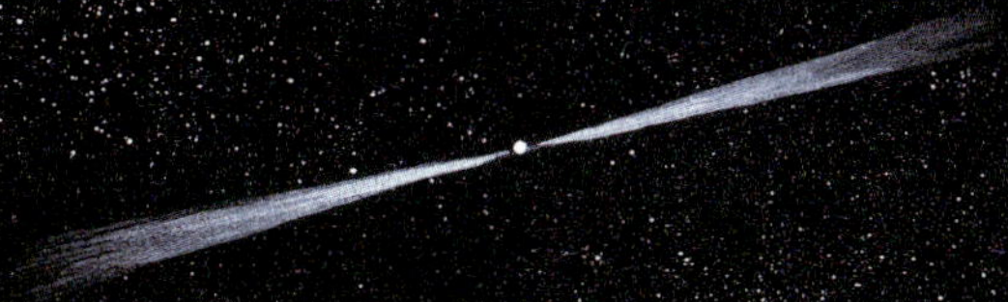

Neutronenstern

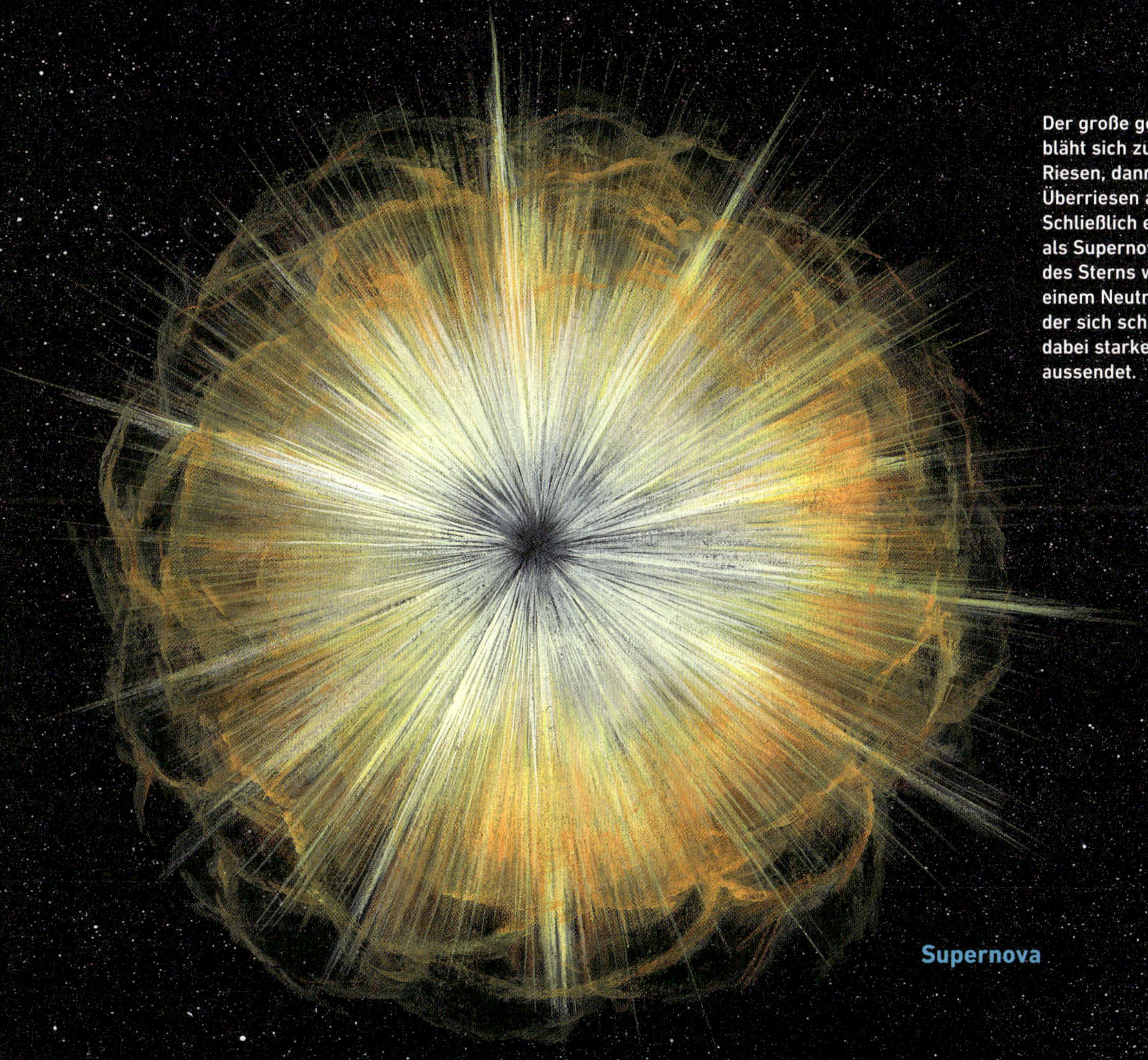

Der große gelbe Stern bläht sich zu einem Roten Riesen, dann zu einem Überriesen auf. Schließlich explodiert er als Supernova. Die Reste des Sterns werden zu einem Neutronenstern, der sich schnell dreht und dabei starke Strahlung aussendet.

Supernova

Woraus besteht die Milchstraße?

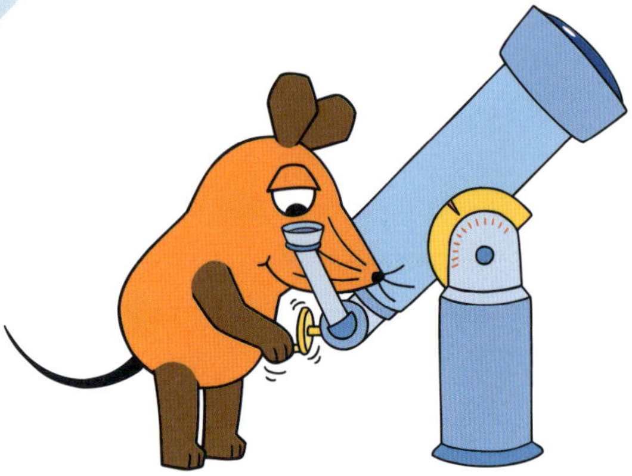

In klaren Nächten sieht man ein helles Band, das sich quer über den Himmel zieht. Wenn du es dir durch ein Teleskop anschaust, kannst du jede Menge einzelne Lichtpunkte erkennen!

Diese Lichtpunkte sind Teil einer gewaltigen Ansammlung von Sternen, zu der auch unsere Sonne gehört. Eine solche Ansammlung von Sternen nennt man **Galaxie**. Unsere Galaxie heißt Milchstraße. Sie sieht aus wie ein Windrad und ist wie eine flache Spirale geformt, mit einer dickeren Stelle in der Mitte.

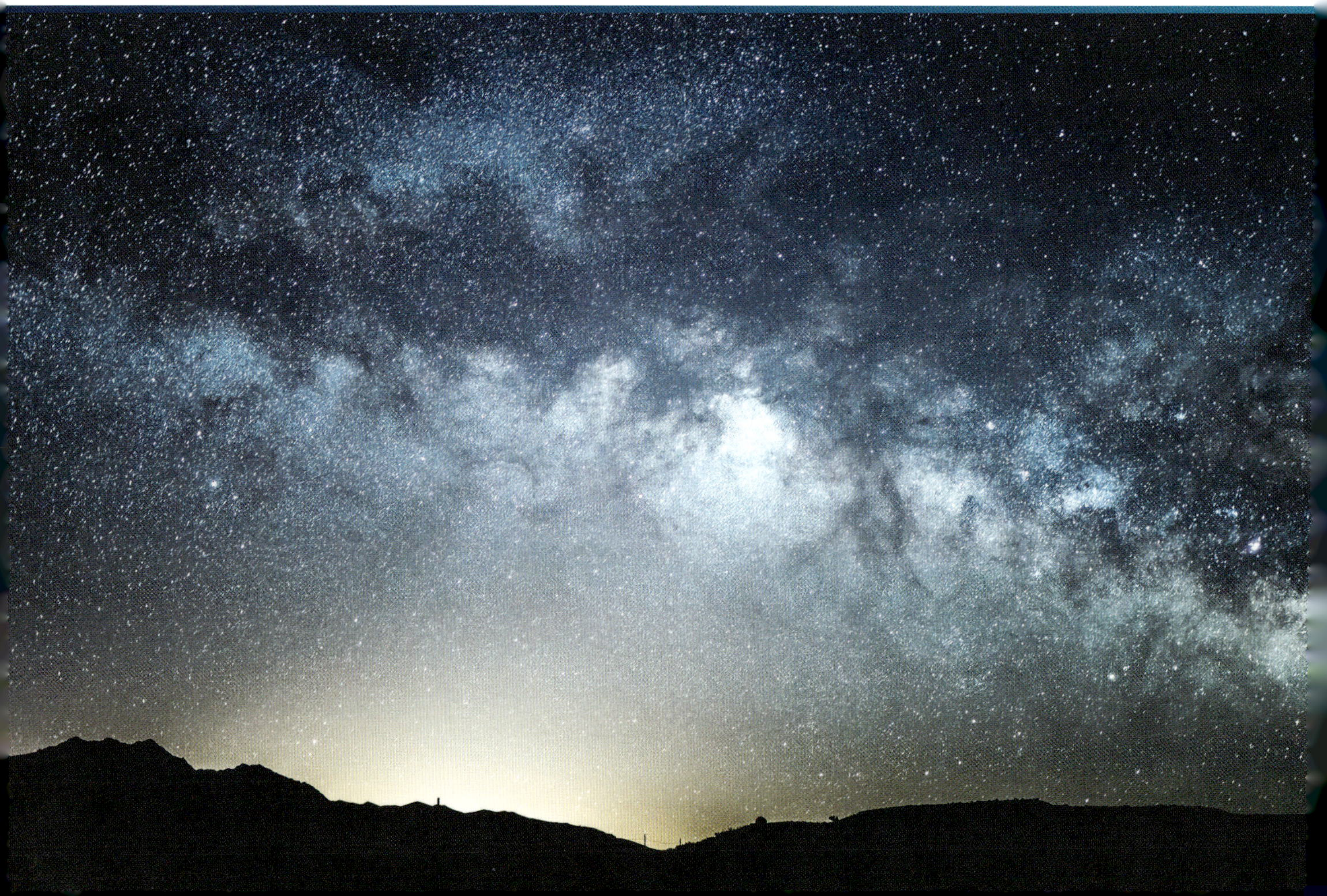

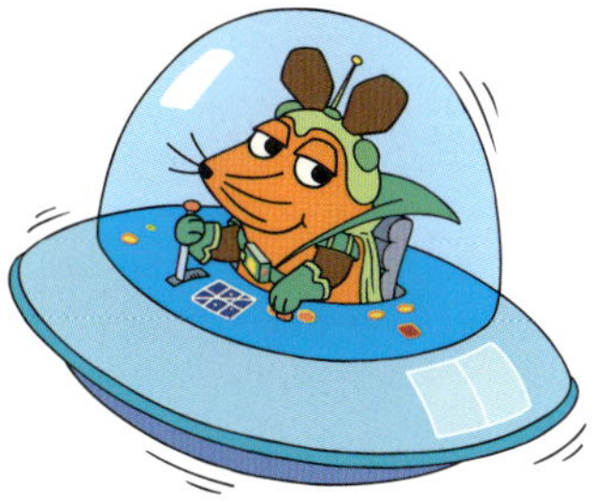

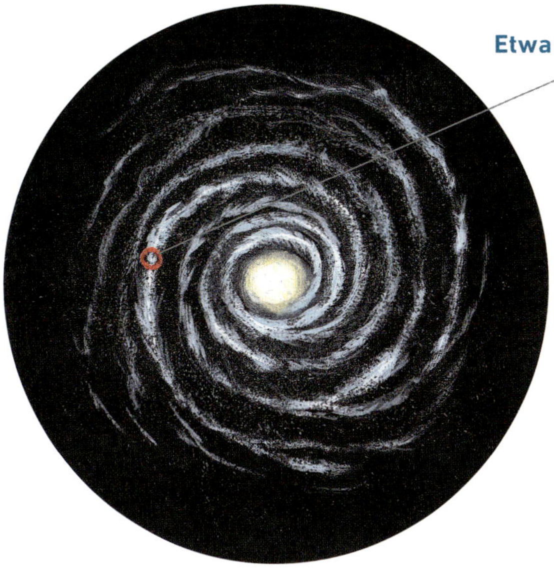

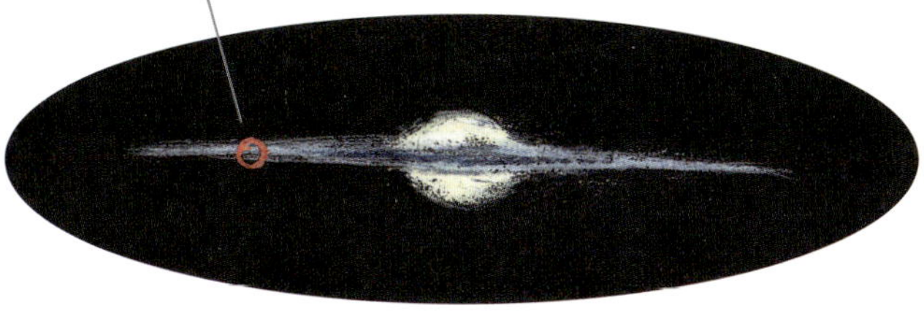
Etwa hier ist unsere Sonne.

Das ist unsere Milchstraße.
Sie ist eine Spiralgalaxie.

Diese Sternenspirale dreht sich und unsere Sonne umkreist die Mitte unserer Galaxie. Aber weil die so riesig ist, braucht die Sonne für jede Runde fast 240 Millionen Jahre.

Außer der **Milchstraße** gibt es viele andere, unterschiedlich geformte Galaxien. Sie kommen meist in Gruppen vor. Unsere Galaxie gehört zur „Lokalen Gruppe". Zu dieser Gruppe gehören etwa 30 Galaxien, allerdings nur zwei richtig große. Wenn wir also einem Außerirdischen unsere Adresse nennen sollten, würden wir sagen: „Dritter Planet der Sonne, Galaxie Milchstraße, Lokale Gruppe".

Unsere Galaxie verschluckt laufend Zwerggalaxien, die durch die Schwerkraft zu ihr hingezogen und somit ein Teil von ihr werden. Und in etwa drei Milliarden Jahren werden die Milchstraße und ihr riesiger Nachbar, die Andromeda-Galaxie, zusammenstoßen. Unserer Sonne wird wahrscheinlich nichts passieren.

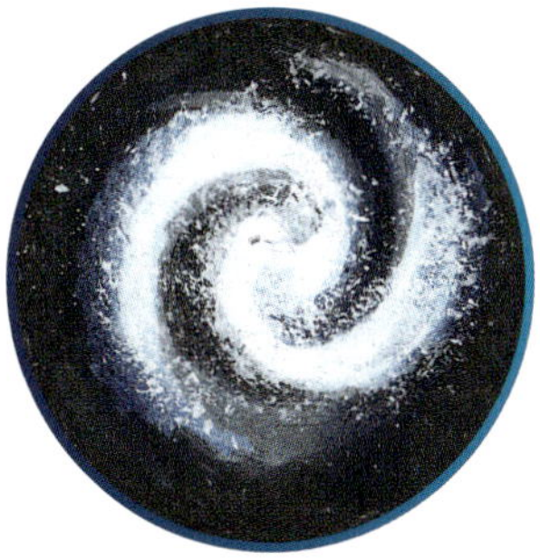

Balkengalaxie

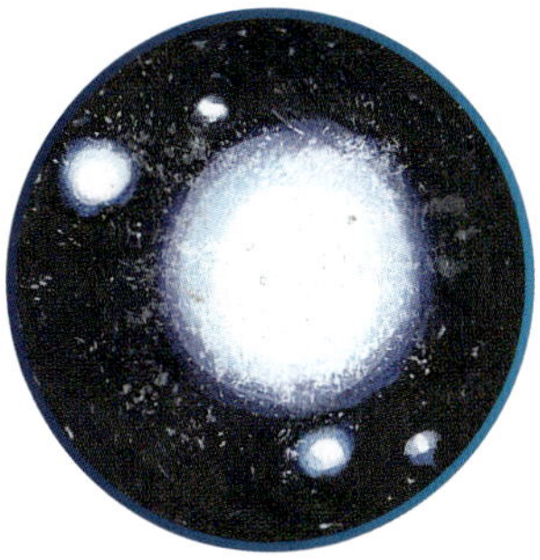

kugelförmige Galaxie

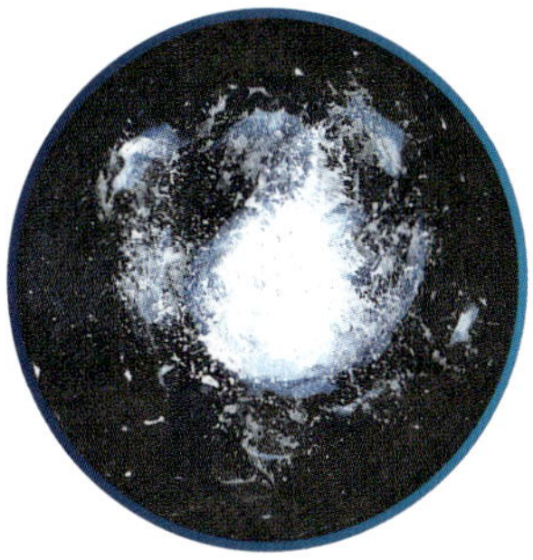

unregelmäßig geformte Galaxie

So unterschiedlich können Galaxien aussehen.

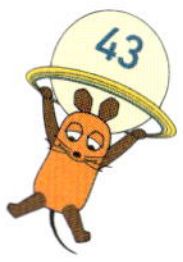

Was ist ein Schwarzes Loch?

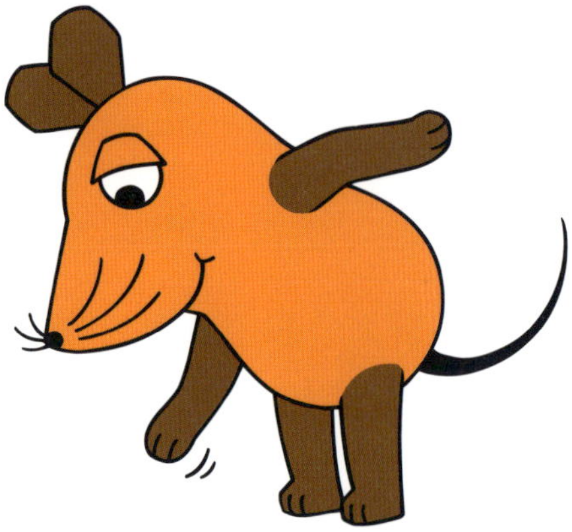

Schwarze Löcher entstehen, wenn ein sehr großer Stern explodiert und ausbrennt. Dieser Stern fällt dann unter seinem eigenen Gewicht zu einem winzigen Punkt zusammen.

Ein Schwarzes Loch sendet aufgrund seiner riesigen **Schwerkraft** kein Licht aus, deshalb ist es so gut wie unsichtbar und sehr schwer zu entdecken. Es ist aber trotzdem sehr gefährlich. Denn es zieht alles in sich hinein, was ihm zu nahe kommt.

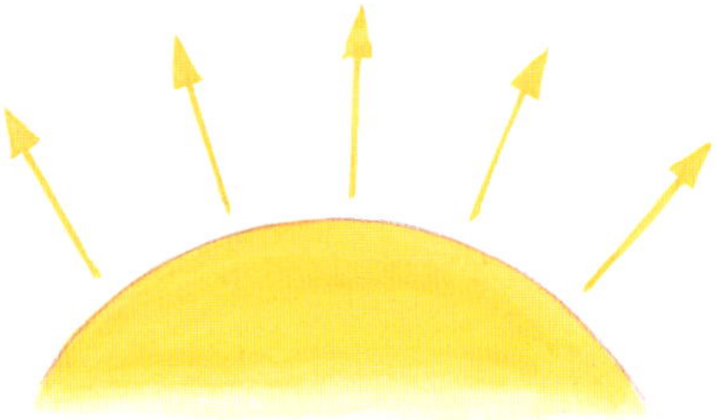

Ein normaler Stern sendet Lichtstrahlen aus.

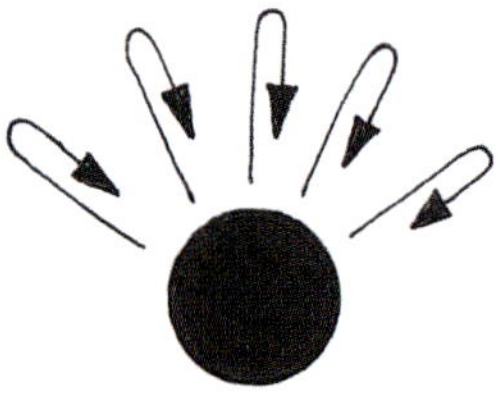

Ein Schwarzes Loch leuchtet nicht, es biegt die Strahlen zu sich selbst zurück.

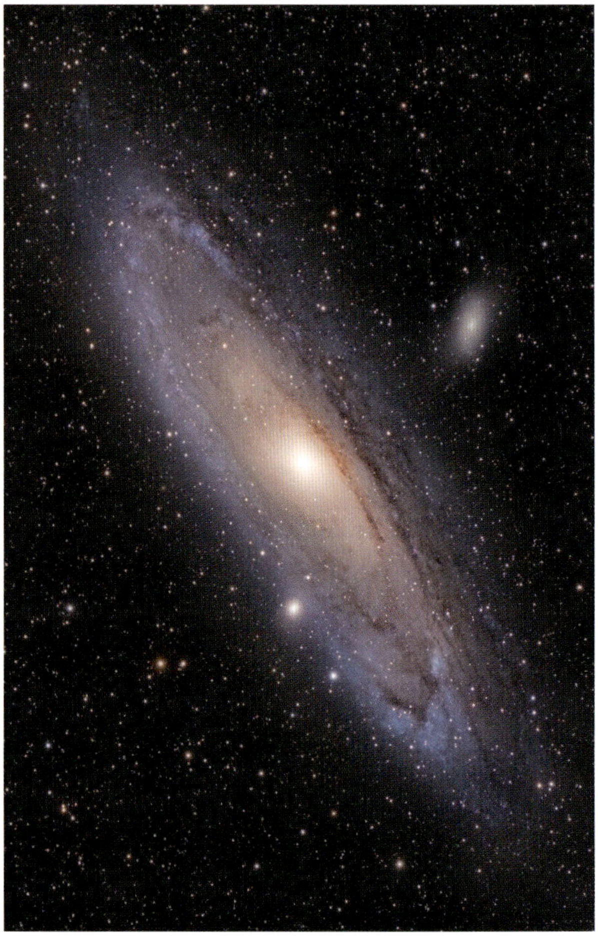

Die Andromeda-Galaxie. Man geht davon aus, dass sich in ihrer Mitte ein riesiges Schwarzes Loch befindet.

Würde man (aus sicherer Entfernung natürlich!) ein Spielzeugauto hineinschubsen, würde die Schwerkraft es zuerst ziemlich in die Länge ziehen. Dann würde es zerrissen und vom Schwarzen Loch in winzige Teilchen und Energie verwandelt werden. Durch diese Teilchen wird der seltsame Himmelskörper jedes Mal ein kleines bisschen dicker und schwerer.

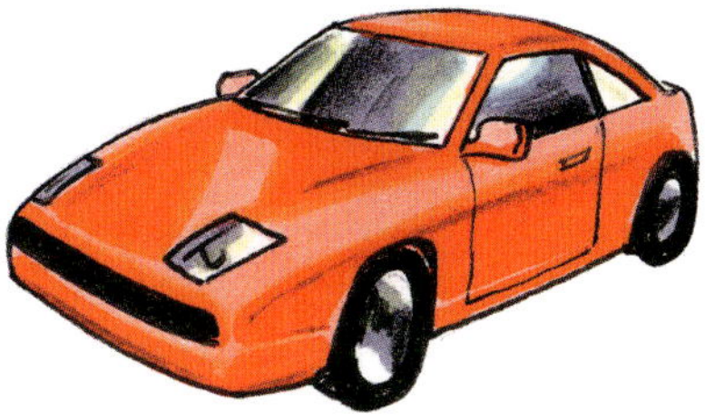

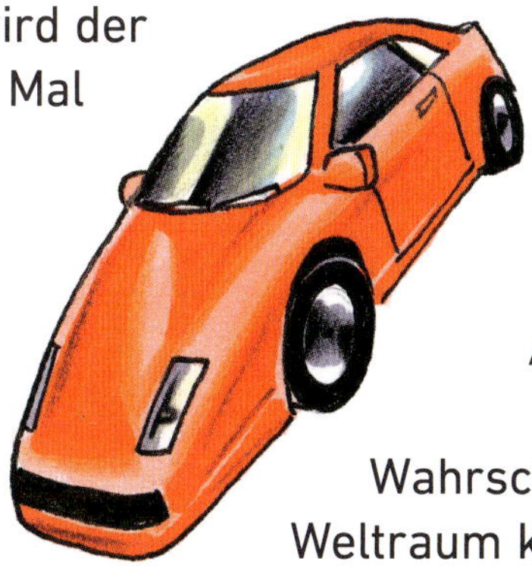

Wie das genau passiert, weiß man noch nicht. Früher dachte man, dass alles, was in ein Schwarzes Loch fällt, für immer verschwindet.

Heute weiß man, dass Dinge nach sehr langer Zeit wieder herauskommen können. Allerdings nur als Teilchen.

Wahrscheinlich gibt es überall im Weltraum kleine und mittelgroße Schwarze Löcher. Soweit man weiß, haben die meisten Galaxien ein besonders großes Schwarzes Loch genau in ihrer Mitte.

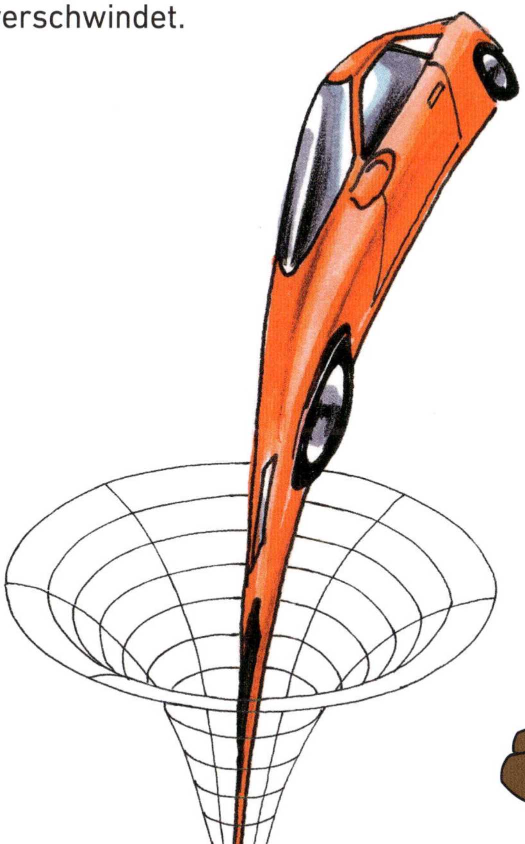

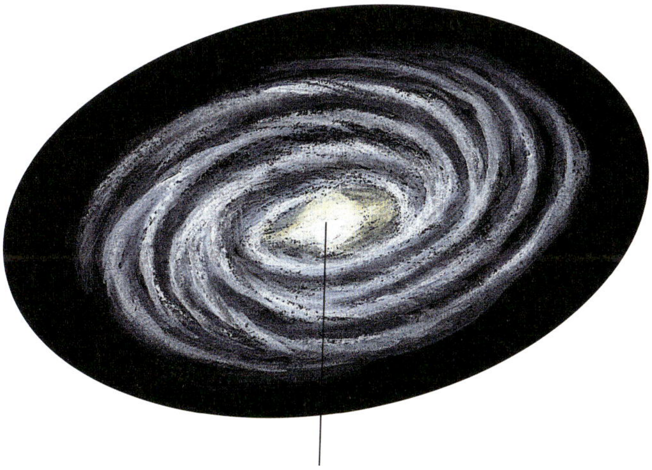

Das Schwarzes Loch befindet sich meist in der Mitte einer Galaxie.

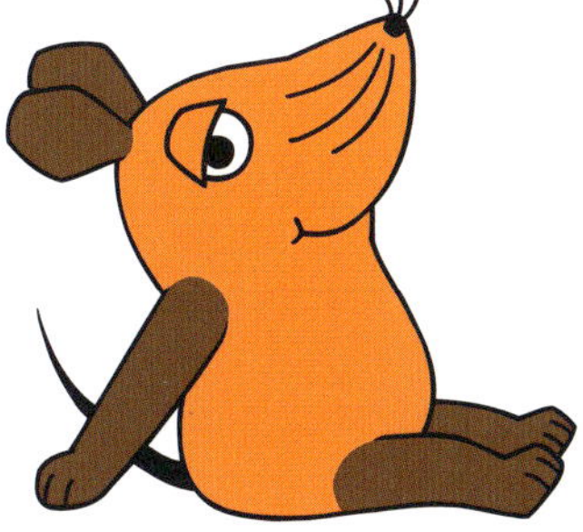

Wie wird man Astronaut?

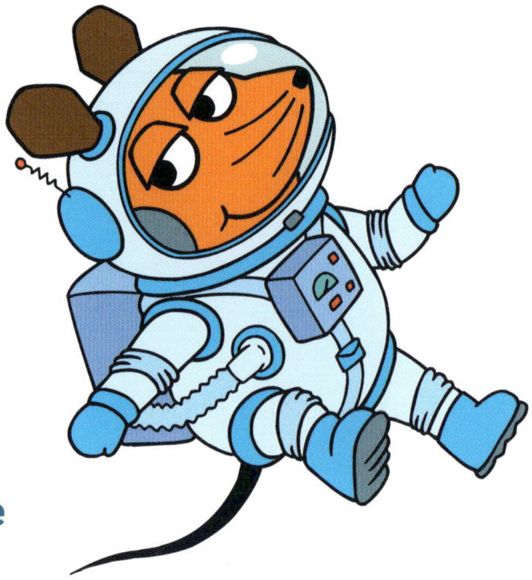

Die ersten Astronauten waren erfahrene Piloten und kamen vom Militär. Heute sucht die europäische Raumfahrtbehörde ESA eher Leute, die Stress aushalten, gut mit anderen Menschen auskommen und Technik oder Naturwissenschaften studiert haben.

An Bord eines **Raumschiffs** oder einer Raumstation arbeiten meist Menschen aus vielen verschiedenen Ländern. Die zukünftigen **Astronauten** bekommen Unterricht in Raumfahrttechnik und Weltraumforschung und erfahren genau, wie die Internationale Raumstation **ISS** funktioniert. Die Schwerelosigkeit lernen sie bei Flügen in einem besonderen Flugzeug kennen.

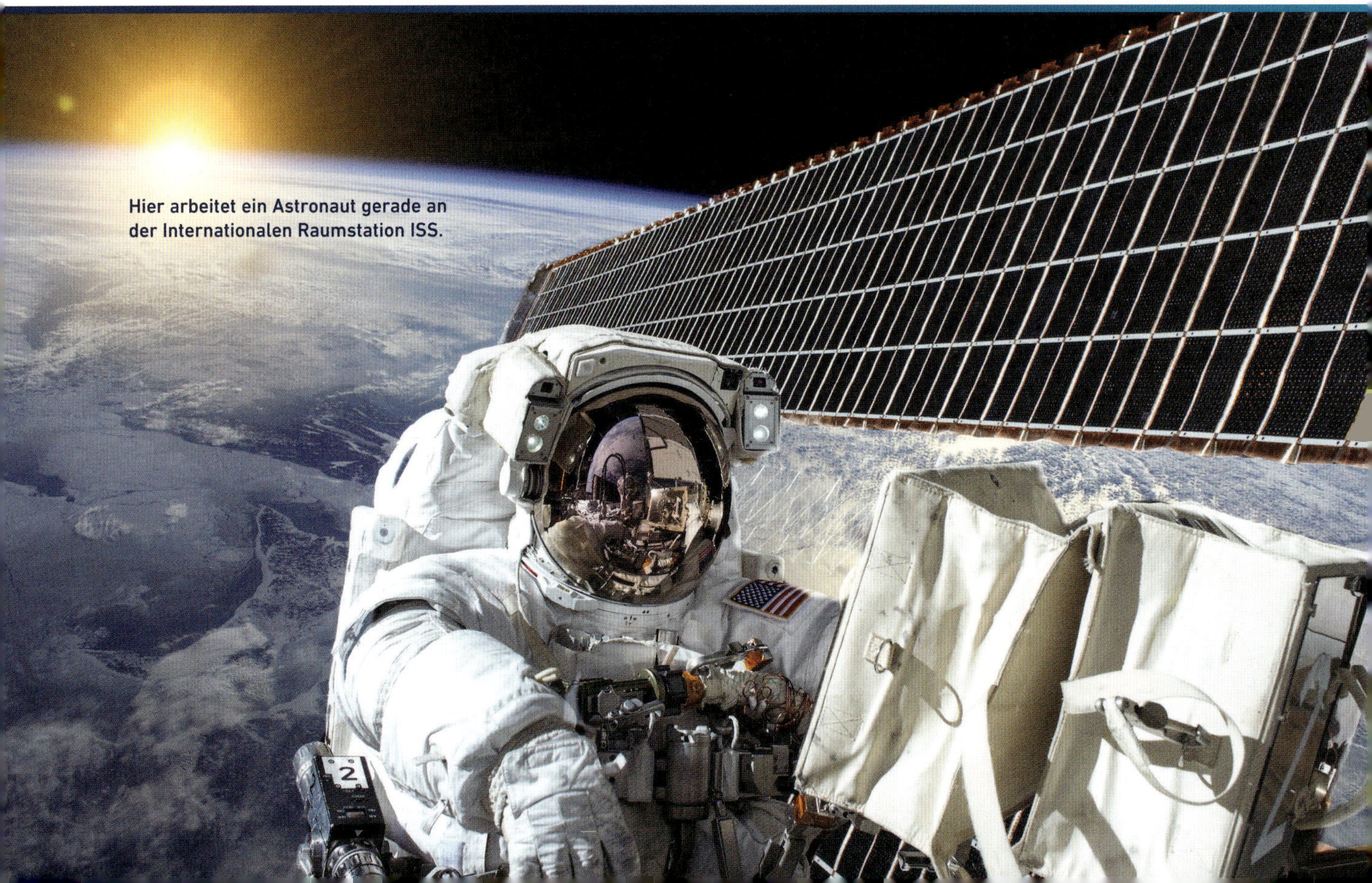

Hier arbeitet ein Astronaut gerade an der Internationalen Raumstation ISS.

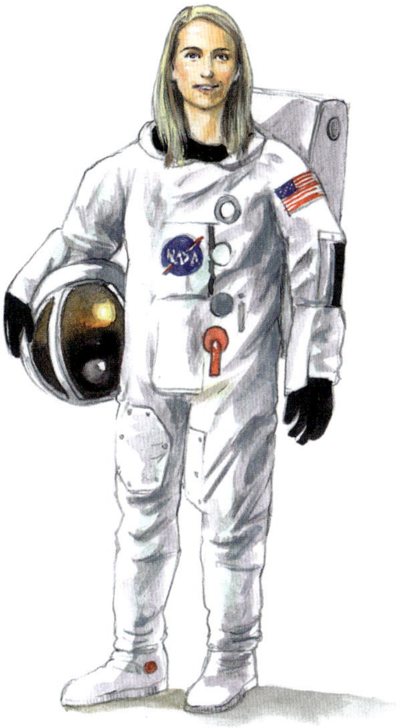

Mit so einem modernen Raumanzug können Astronauten im Weltall spazieren gehen.

In Tauchbecken fühlt man sich ebenfalls schwerelos. Hier üben die **Astronauten**, Reparaturen durchzuführen. Sie trainieren genau die Aufgaben, die sie bei ihrem Flug erwarten. Denn bei jedem Flug werden andere wissenschaftliche Experimente gemacht.

Drei bis sieben Monate sind die Astronauten zu dritt auf der Internationalen Raumstation. Dort sind sie sehr viel mit Experimenten und Arbeiten an der Station beschäftigt und haben eine tolle Aussicht auf die Erde. Duschen können sie nicht, weil das Wasser in der Schwerelosigkeit immer wegschweben würde. Deswegen müssen sie sich mit feuchten Tüchern waschen.

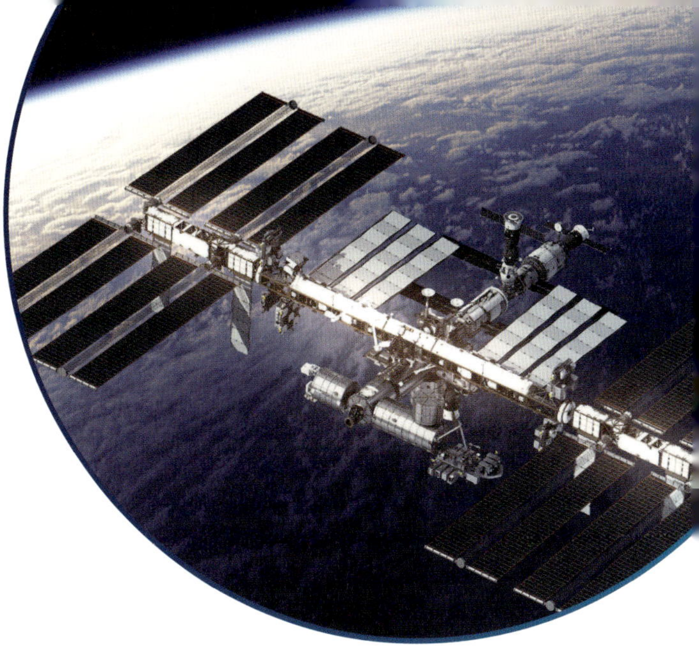

Wenn sie schlafen wollen, befestigen sie ihren Schlafsack irgendwo an der Wand oder Decke, kriechen hinein und machen die Augen zu.

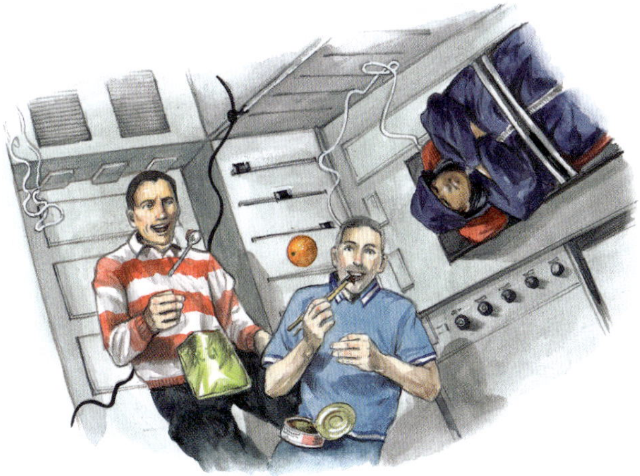

An Bord einer Raumstation müssen die Astronauten aufpassen, dass ihnen das Essen nicht davonfliegt.

Auf der ISS gibt es besondere Toiletten. Das große oder kleine Geschäft wird sofort abgesaugt.

Wie funktionieren eine Rakete und ein Raumschiff?

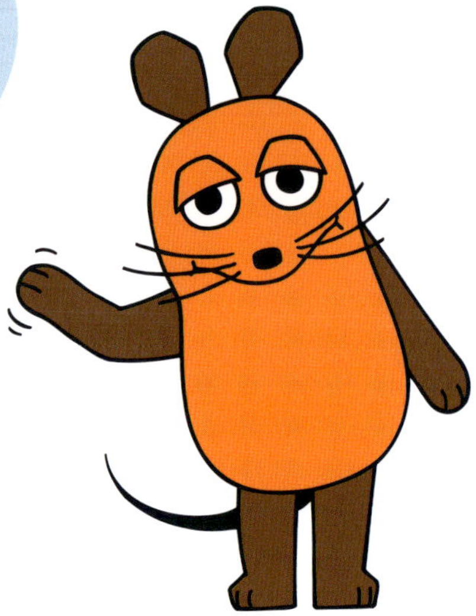

Raketen und Raumschiffe werden von den Gasen angeschoben, die sie ausstoßen. Das ist, wie wenn du einen Luftballon aufbläst und die Öffnung zuhältst. Wenn du ihn loslässt, zischt Luft aus dem Ballon heraus und er fliegt weg.

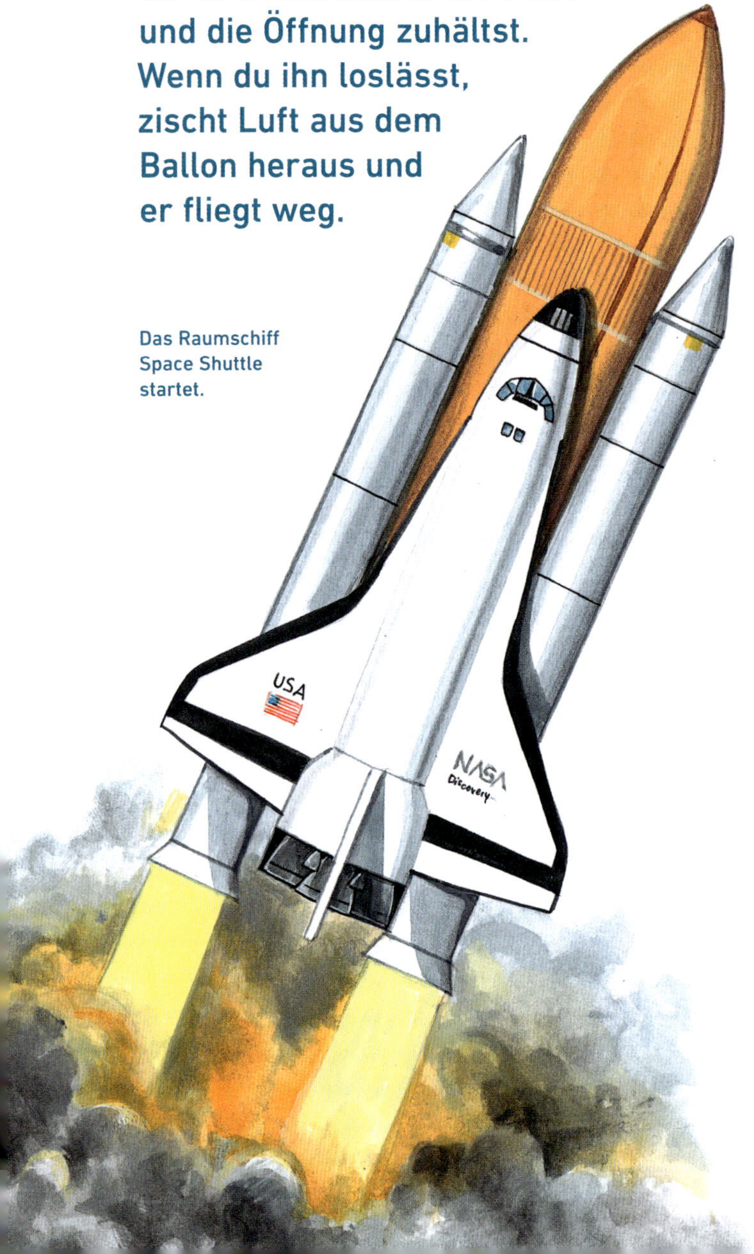

Das Raumschiff Space Shuttle startet.

Es gibt zwei unterschiedliche Arten von Raumfahrzeugen:

1. **Raumschiffe** sind Fahrzeuge mit Menschen an Bord, die mehrmals in den Weltraum fliegen und wieder zurückkommen können.
2. **Raketen** sind längliche Raumfahrzeuge, die man nur einmal benutzen kann. Mit ihnen kann man etwas von der Erde in den Weltraum bringen.

Beide Raumfahrzeuge lassen sich beim Start von zwei an den Seiten angebrachten Raketen, die man **Booster** nennt, anschieben. Sie sind mit einem festen Brennstoff gefüllt. Wenn er entzündet wird und abbrennt, entstehen große Mengen heißes Gas, das schnell ausströmt. Nach ein paar Minuten sind die Booster ausgebrannt, werden abgeworfen und stürzen ins Meer.

Das ist die Rakete Ariane. An ihren Seiten sind die beiden Booster zu sehen.

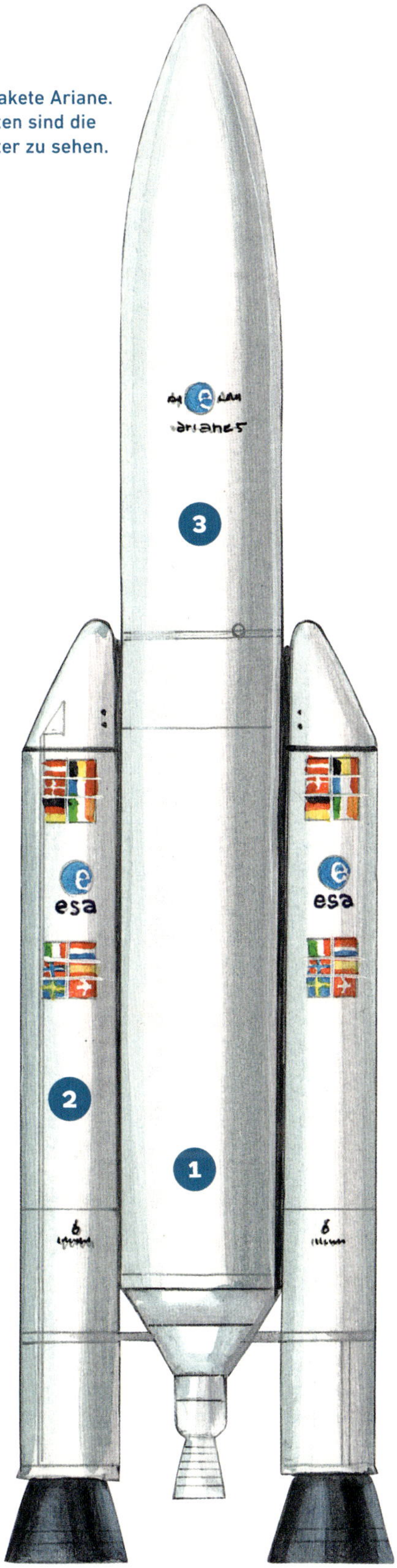

1 Haupttriebwerk

2 Booster

3 Obere Raketenstufe

Nun übernimmt das Haupt-**Triebwerk**, das mit flüssigem Treibstoff funktioniert. Das Raumschiff hat einen riesigen Extra-Tank dabei, weil es so viel Treibstoff verbraucht. Wenn dieser leer ist, wird auch er abgeworfen. Inzwischen ist das Raumschiff so hoch geflogen, dass es nicht mehr auf die Erde zurückfällt, sondern sie etwa alle neunzig Minuten einmal umkreist. Mit einer Art Greifarm heben die Astronauten die Dinge heraus, die das Raumschiff mitgebracht hat. Zum Beispiel einen **Satelliten**, einen kleinen Flugkörper, der bestimmte Aufgaben erfüllen kann.

Eine Rakete kann mit ihrer zweiten Raketenstufe noch höher fliegen. Wenn ihre **Satelliten** ausgesetzt sind, hat die Rakete ihre Aufgabe erfüllt. Ihre Reste bleiben im Weltall. Ein Raumschiff kehrt nach einigen Wochen zurück zur Erde und landet dort ähnlich wie ein Flugzeug.

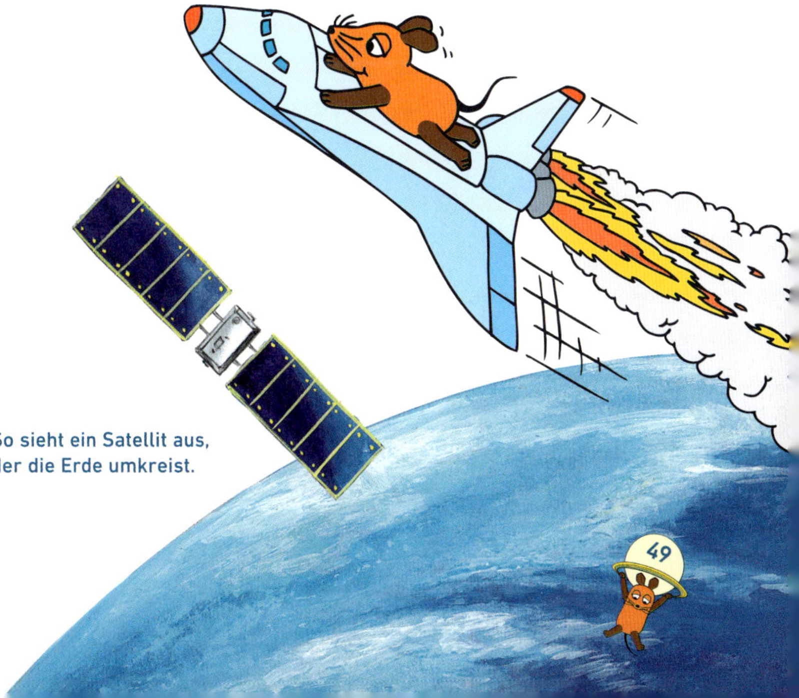

So sieht ein Satellit aus, der die Erde umkreist.

Wie lange fliegt man zum Mond?

Um zum Mond zu fliegen, brauchst du ein Raumschiff. Der Flug dauert etwa drei Tage.

Raumkapsel und Mondfähre fliegen weiter zum Mond.

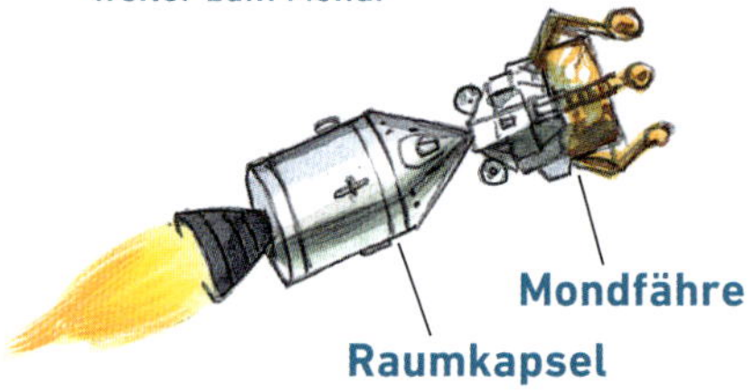

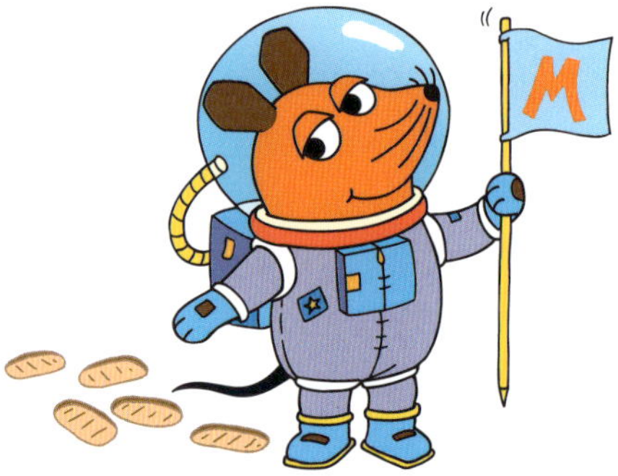

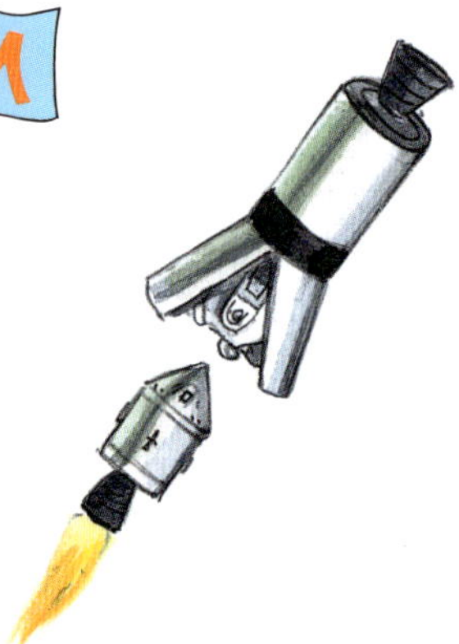

Die Raumkapsel verbindet sich mit der Mondfähre. Die Rakete wird abgetrennt.

In den 1960er-Jahren waren die USA mit der Sowjetunion (die heute Russland heißt) verfeindet. Beide Länder wollten sich ständig beweisen, dass sie besser sind. Die Sowjetunion schaffte es, den allerersten Satelliten und den ersten Menschen in den Weltraum zu bringen. Die USA wollten nun wenigstens den ersten Menschen auf dem Mond abset-zen. Dafür bauten sie eine 111 Meter hohe Rakete, die Saturn V. Mit fast 40.000 Stundenkilometern beförderte die Rakete das „Apollo 11" getaufte Raumschiff mit drei Astronauten an Bord Richtung Mond. Ein Kontrollzent-rum auf der Erde überwachte den Flug.

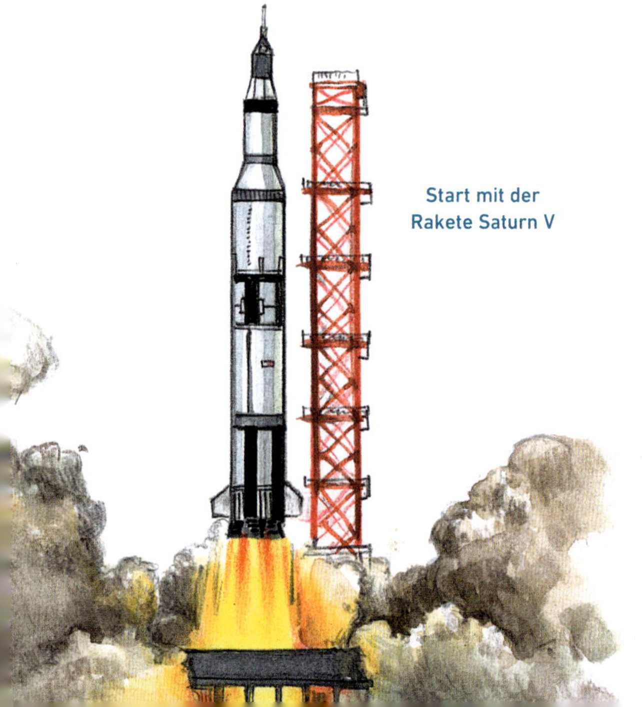

Start mit der Rakete Saturn V

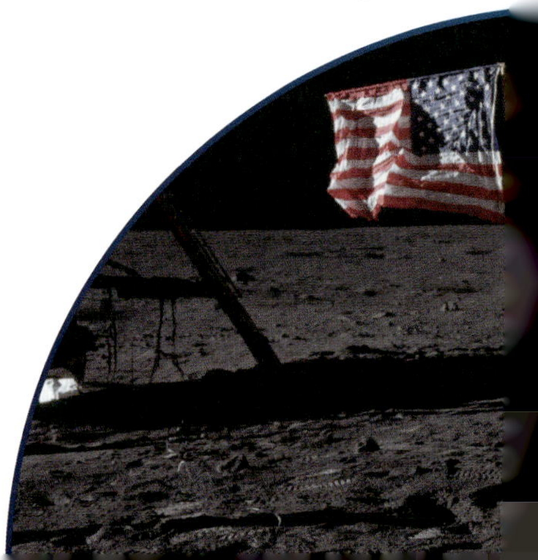

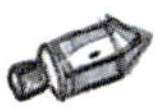

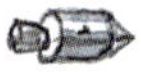

Zwei Astronauten landen mit der Mondfähre und erkunden den Landeplatz.

Dann fliegen sie wieder zurück zur Raumkapsel. Dabei lassen sie einen Teil der Mondfähre auf dem Mond zurück.

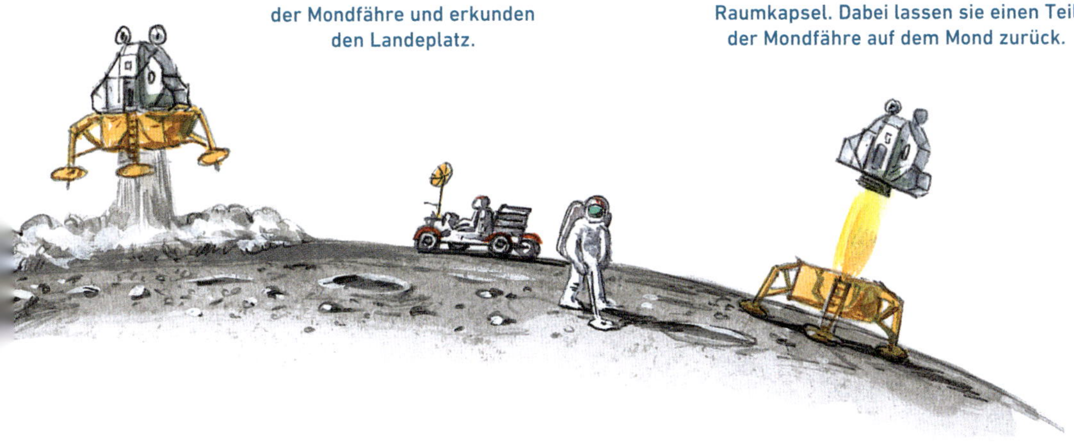

Die Mondfähre dockt wieder an der Raumkapsel an.

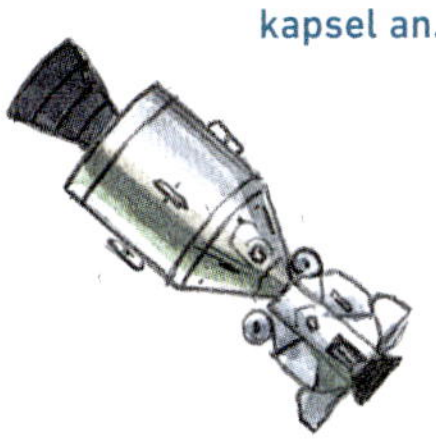

Da es auf dem Mond keine Luft gibt, trugen die **Astronauten** Raumanzüge und atmeten einen Luftvorrat, den sie mitgebracht hatten. Da die **Schwerkraft** des Mondes schwächer ist als die der Erde, konnten die **Astronauten** bei ihrem Spaziergang ohne Mühe zweieinhalb Meter weit springen.

Armstrong und die anderen schafften es wieder zurück auf die Erde. Nach ihnen landeten noch zehn Amerikaner auf dem Mond. Seit 1972 war niemand mehr auf dem Mond – aber das soll sich bald wieder ändern.

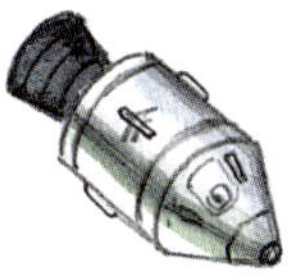

Die Astronauten steigen in die Raumkapsel um und fliegen zurück zur Erde.

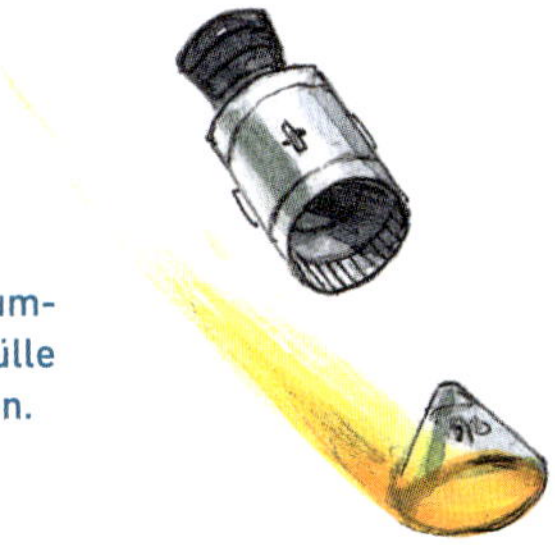

Nur die Spitze der Raumkapsel kann die Lufthülle der Erde durchqueren.

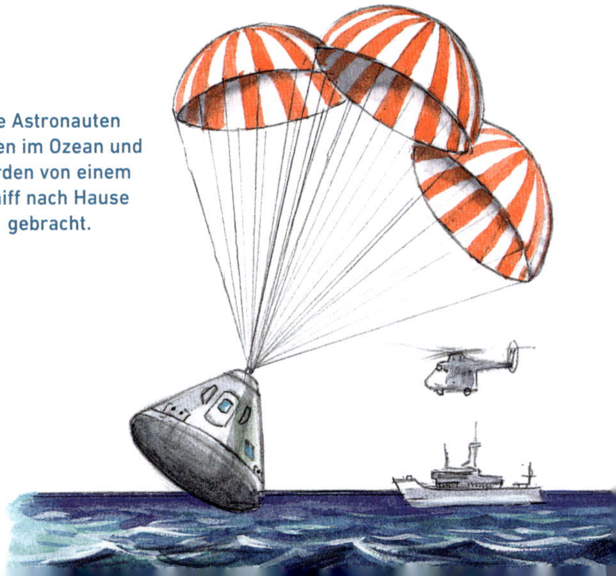

Die Astronauten landen im Ozean und werden von einem Schiff nach Hause gebracht.

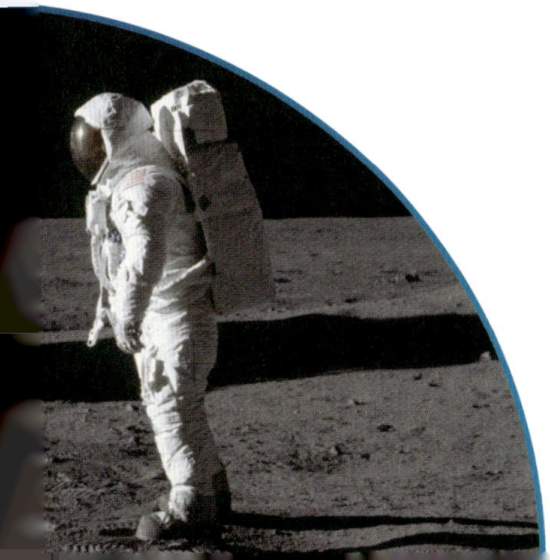

Am 21. Juli 1969 betraten Neil Armstrong und Edwin Aldrin als erste Menschen den Mond. Sie stellten dort eine amerikanische Flagge auf.

Wann kann man im Weltraum Urlaub machen?

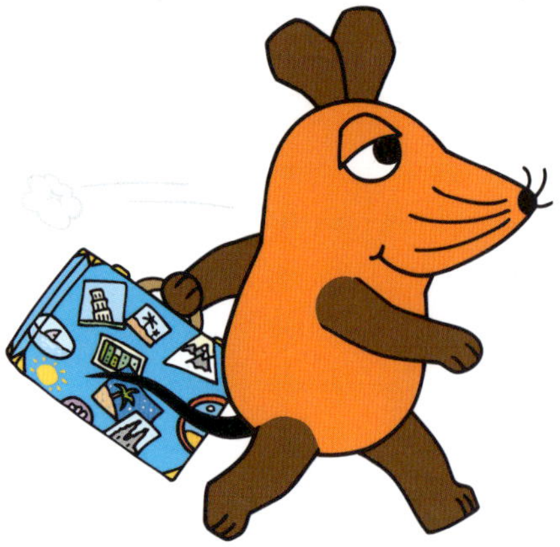

Das ist jetzt schon möglich. Im Moment ist ein Touristenflug in den Weltraum allerdings sehr teuer. Mindestens 20 Millionen Dollar (also etwa 17,5 Millionen Euro) pro Person kostet es, mal auf der Raumstation ISS vorbeizuschauen! Doch es kann sein, dass Weltraumflüge bald billiger werden.

Erfinder und Unternehmen in aller Welt arbeiten daran, kleine Raumschiffe für Touristenflüge zu entwickeln. Das Ziel ist es, ohne die Hilfe der großen Raumfahrtbehörden in den Weltraum zu kommen. Einige Unternehmen wollen Rundflüge um die Erde anbieten, andere planen sogar Reisen bis zum Mond. Den ersten privat finanzierten Weltraumflug hat 2004 eine amerikanische Firma durchgeführt. Ihr „SpaceShipOne" kam auf über 100 Kilometer Höhe, das gilt schon als Weltraum. Aber bis wir den Urlaub auf dem Mond im Reisebüro buchen können, wird es wohl noch eine Weile dauern.

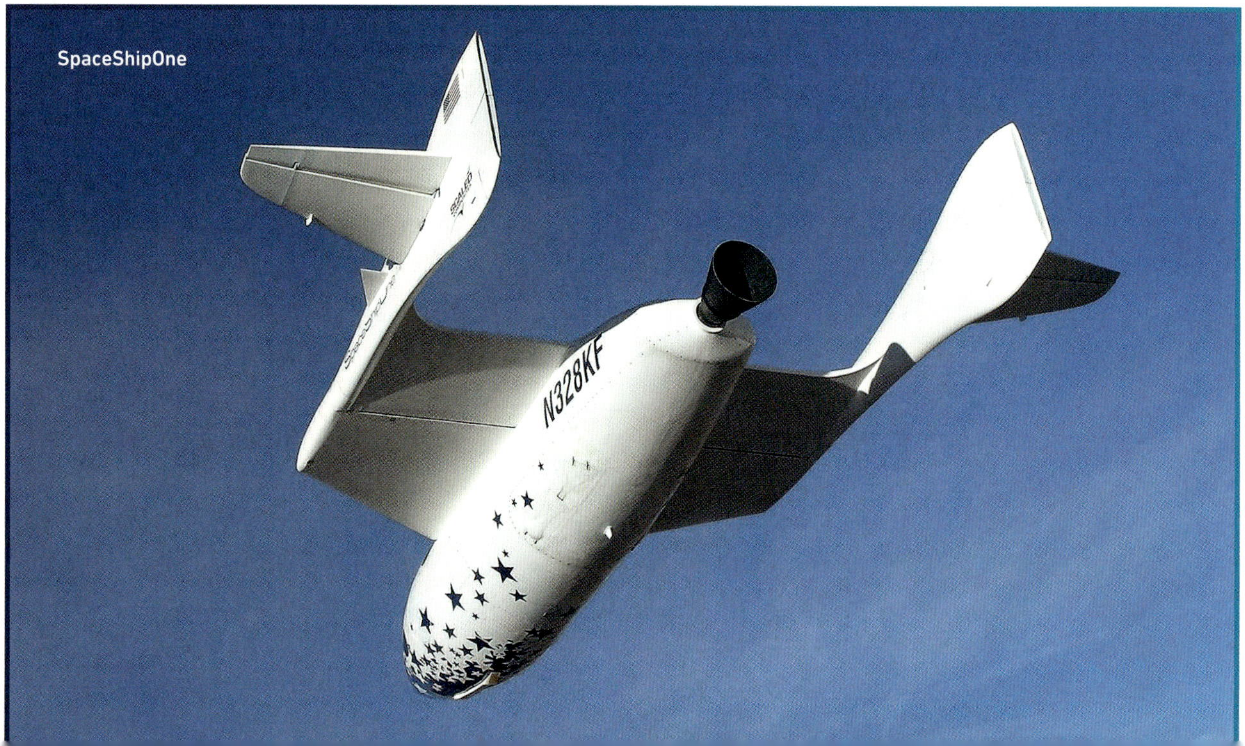

SpaceShipOne

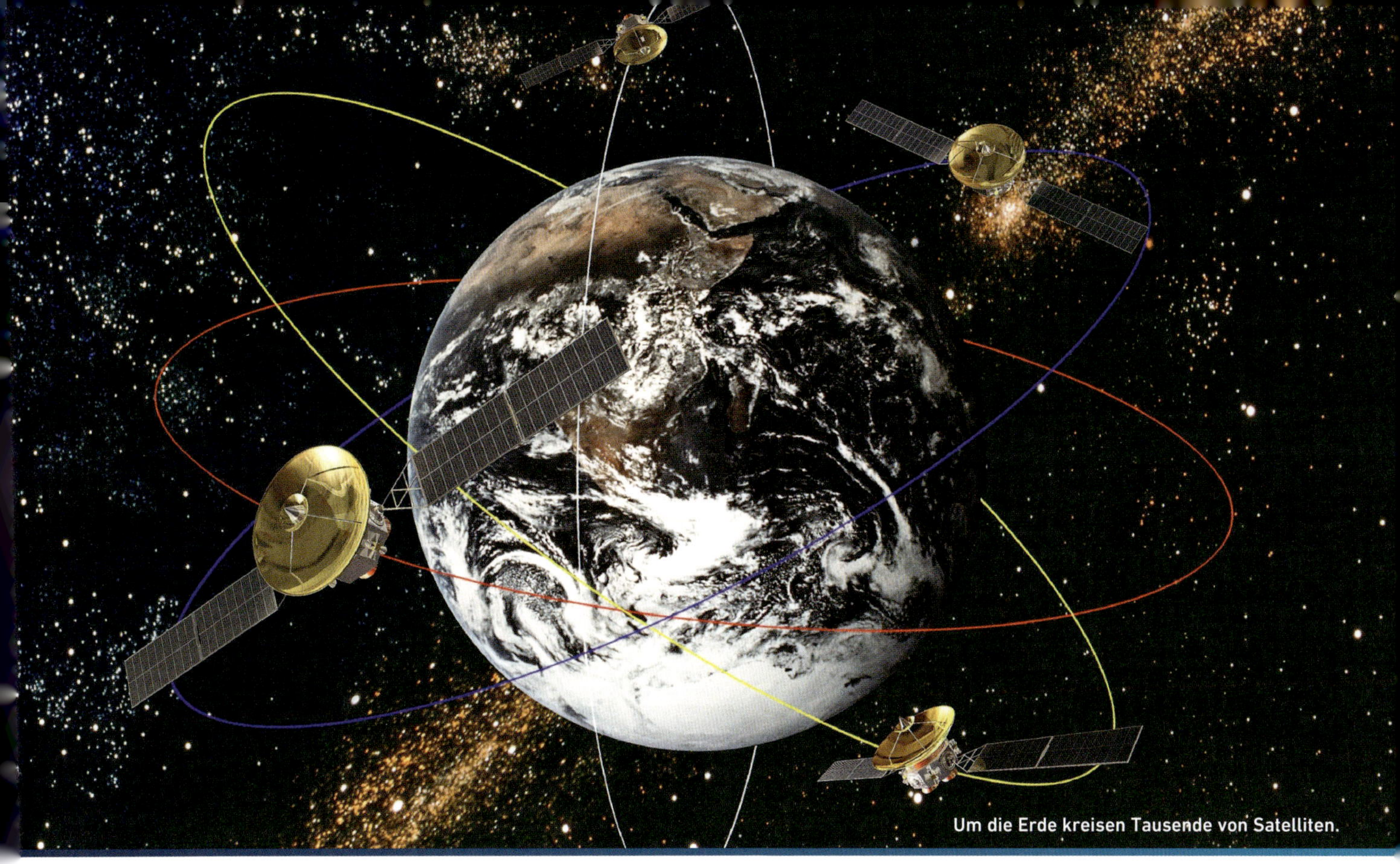

Um die Erde kreisen Tausende von Satelliten.

Ganz ungefährlich ist so ein Flug ins All nicht. Zum Beispiel könnte ein Stück **Weltraummüll** auf das **Raumschiff** prallen, mit dem du gerade in den Urlaub fliegst. Dieser Müll ist ein echtes Problem geworden. Er besteht vor allem aus Tausenden von alten und kaputten **Satelliten**, die noch immer um die Erde kreisen.

Hinzu kommen ausgebrannte Teile von Raketen und Dreck, der aus Raumschiffen über Bord geworfen wurde. Viele Wissenschaftler machen sich darüber Gedanken, wie man diesen Schrott wieder los wird.

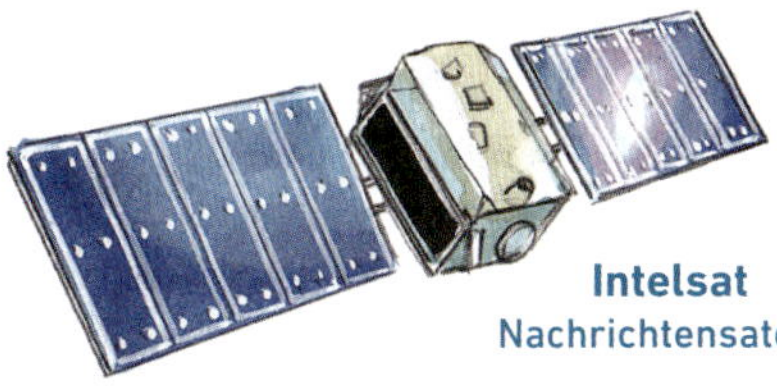

Intelsat
Nachrichtensatellit

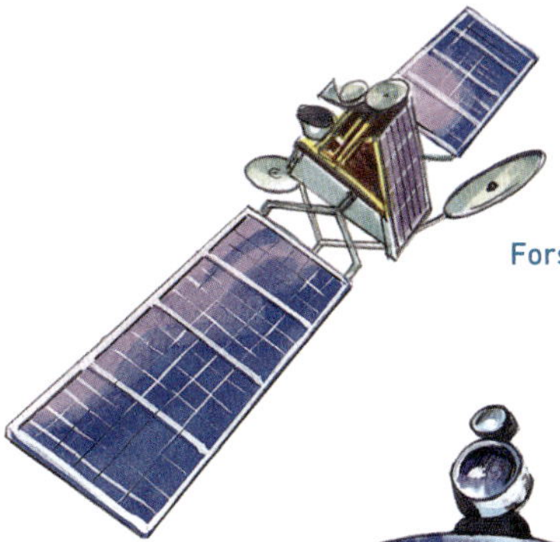

Eureka
Forschungssatellit

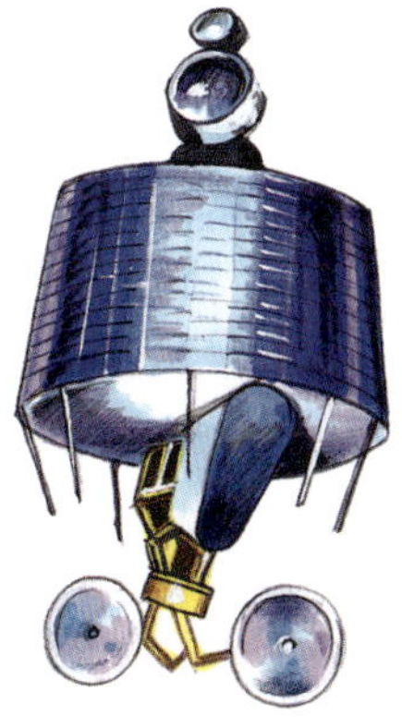

Himawari
Wettersatellit

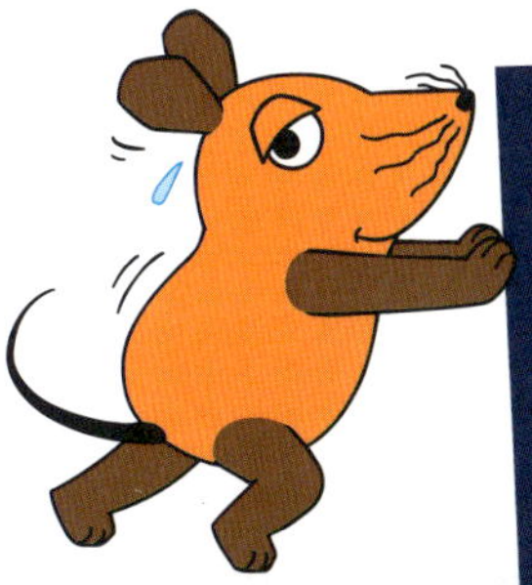

Satelliten dienen zum Beispiel dazu, das Wetter zu überwachen oder Daten und Telefongespräche weiterzuleiten. Sie umkreisen die Erde ohne Menschen an Bord.

Mauslexikon

Äquator: Gedachte Linie um die Erde herum. Sie ist von Nord- und Südpol gleich weit entfernt und teilt die Erdkugel in eine Nord- und eine Südhalbkugel.

Asteroidengürtel: Ring aus Gesteinsbrocken, der zwischen Mars und Jupiter um die Sonne kreist.

Astronaut: Teilnehmer eines Weltraumfluges. In Russland nennt man diese Raumfahrer auch Kosmonauten, in China Taikonauten.

Astronom: Wissenschaftler, der sich mit Sternen und Planeten beschäftigt.

Booster: Mit festem Treibstoff gefüllte Teile eines Raumschiffs oder einer Rakete, die beim Start gebraucht werden. Einmal gezündet, brennen sie so lange, bis sie leer sind; man kann sie nicht abschalten.

Fliehkraft: Kraft, die auf einen Körper wirkt, der sich kreisförmig bewegt. Sie drängt den Körper nach außen.

Galaxie: Gigantische Ansammlung von Sternen.

ISS: Abkürzung für „International Space Station". Das ist der Name der Internationalen Raumstation.

Kuiper-Gürtel: Ring aus Gesteinsbrocken, der hinter dem Neptun um die Sonne kreist.

Meteor: Fachbegriff für Sternschnuppe. Leuchtstreifen am Himmel. Er stammt von einem kleinen Stein oder Staubkorn aus dem Weltraum, das gerade in der Lufthülle der Erde verglüht.

Meteorit: Steinbrocken aus dem Weltraum, der auf die Erde gestürzt ist.

Milchstraße: Name der Galaxie, in der wir leben. Die Galaxie Milchstraße hat die Form einer Spirale.

Mondfinsternis: Der Mond wandert durch den großen Schatten der Erde und sieht dadurch dunkler aus.

Neutronenstern: Rest eines großen Sterns, dem der Brennstoff ausgegangen ist.

Planet: Großer Himmelskörper aus Gestein oder Gas, der mit seiner Schwerkraft seine Umgebung beherrscht und oft einen oder mehrere Monde hat.

Raumanzug: Anzug der Astronauten. Mit ihm kann man sich im Weltraum bewegen, wo es sehr kalt oder sehr heiß ist und es keine Luft gibt.

Raumsonde: Weltraumfahrzeug, das dazu dient, Planeten oder andere Himmelskörper zu erforschen.

Satellit: Kleiner Raumflugkörper ohne Personen darin. Wird von einem Raumschiff oder einer Rakete in eine kreisförmige Bahn um die Erde gebracht.

Schallwellen: Geräusche bestehen aus Schallwellen, die sich unsichtbar durch die Luft bewegen. Wenn sie auf deine Ohren treffen, hörst du etwas.

Schwarzes Loch: Himmelskörper, der entsteht, wenn ein sehr großer Stern stirbt. Hat eine sehr starke Schwerkraft und ist fast unsichtbar.

Schwerkraft: Kraft, die jeder Himmelskörper besitzt – je größer er ist, desto stärker ist seine Schwerkraft. Die Schwerkraft zieht alles in der Umgebung zu diesem Himmelskörper hin.

Sonnenfinsternis: Der Mond schiebt sich zwischen Sonne und Erde. Dadurch verdeckt er ein paar Minuten lang die Sonne.

Sonnensystem: So nennt man unsere Sonne und ihre Planeten.

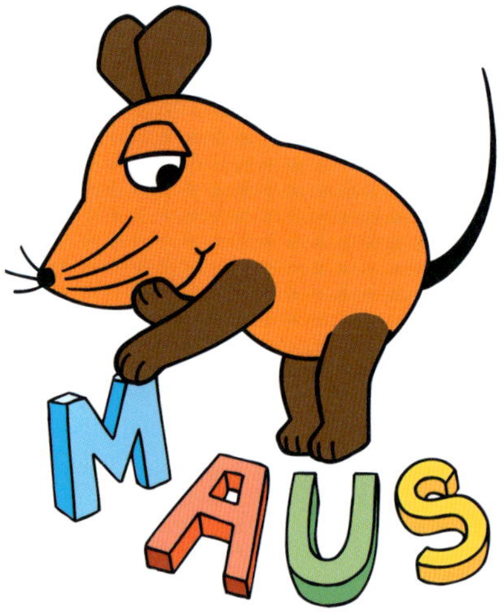

Stern: Riesiger leuchtender Himmelskörper aus glühendem Gas.

Supernova: Stern, der seinen Brennstoff verbraucht hat und deswegen explodiert. Für kurze Zeit ist eine Supernova unglaublich hell, ein paar Tage später ist nur noch ein riesiger Nebel übrig.

Teleskop: Anderes Wort für Fernrohr. Ein längliches Gerät, durch das man Sterne und Planeten stark vergrößert sieht.

Triebwerk: Motor eines Raumschiffs.

Umlaufbahn: Flugbahn eines Himmelskörpers oder Raumschiffs um einen Planeten, Mond oder Stern herum. Meist kreisförmig oder elliptisch (eiförmig).

Universum: Anderes Wort für Weltall.

Weißer Zwerg: Rest eines Sterns, dem der Brennstoff ausgegangen ist. Der Weiße Zwerg kühlt im Laufe von Milliarden Jahren immer stärker ab, bis er ganz erlischt und zu einem Schwarzen Zwerg wird.

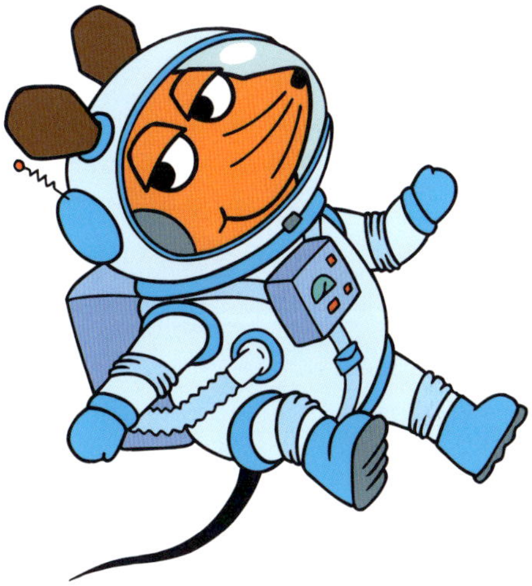

Register

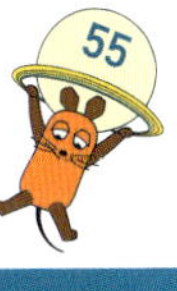

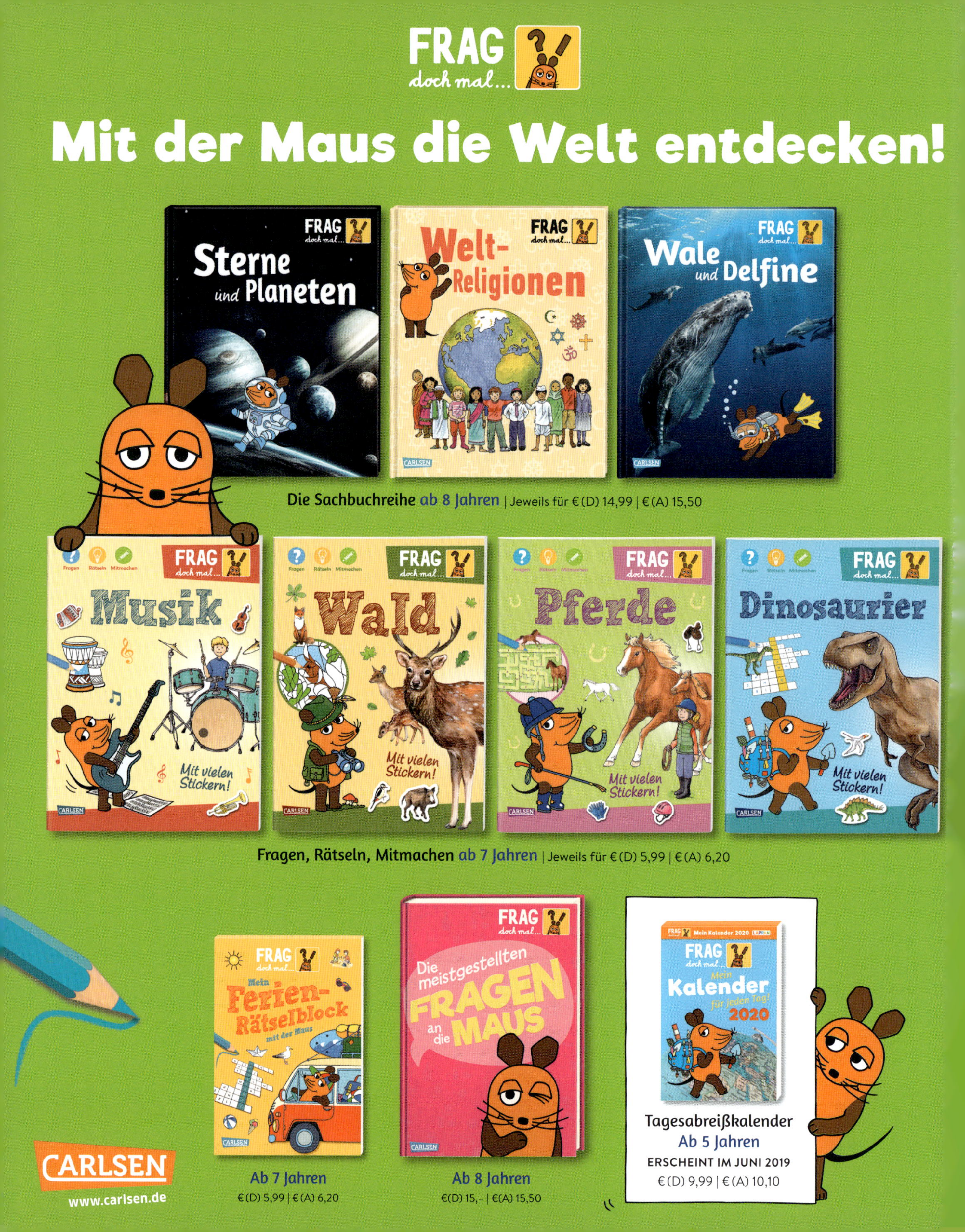
FRAG doch mal …
Mit der Maus die Welt entdecken!
FRAG doch mal … Sterne und Planeten
FRAG doch mal … Welt-Religionen
FRAG doch mal … Wale und Delfine
Die Sachbuchreihe ab 8 Jahren | Jeweils für € (D) 14,99 | € (A) 15,50
FRAG doch mal … Musik Mit vielen Stickern!
FRAG doch mal … Wald Mit vielen Stickern!
FRAG doch mal … Pferde Mit vielen Stickern!
FRAG doch mal … Dinosaurier Mit vielen Stickern!
Fragen, Rätseln, Mitmachen ab 7 Jahren | Jeweils für € (D) 5,99 | € (A) 6,20
FRAG doch mal … Mein Ferien-Rätselblock mit der Maus
Ab 7 Jahren
€ (D) 5,99 | € (A) 6,20
FRAG doch mal … Die meistgestellten FRAGEN an die MAUS
Ab 8 Jahren
€ (D) 15,– | € (A) 15,50
FRAG doch mal … Mein Kalender für jeden Tag! 2020
Tagesabreißkalender
Ab 5 Jahren
ERSCHEINT IM JUNI 2019
€ (D) 9,99 | € (A) 10,10
CARLSEN
www.carlsen.de